The Objective Structured Clinical Examination in ANAESTHESIA

Practice papers for teachers and trainees

Cyprian Mendonca MD FRCA
Shyam Balasubramanian MD FRCA

tfm Publishing Limited, Castle Hill Barns, Harley, Nr Shrewsbury, SY5 6LX, UK. Tel: +44 (0)1952 510061; Fax: +44 (0)1952 510192 E-mail: nikki@tfmpublishing.com; Web site: www.tfmpublishing.com

Design & Typesetting: Nikki Bramhill, tfm publishing Ltd.
First Edition: © September 2007
Background cover image © Comstock Inc., www.comstock.com

ISBN: 978 1 903378 56 4

Printed by Gutenberg Press Ltd., Gudja Road, Tarxien, PLA 19, Malta. Tel: +356 21897037; Fax: +356 21800069.

Contents

OSCE set 2

OSCE set 3

OSCE set 4

OSCE set 5

Preface

The aim of this book is to help trainees sitting the primary fellowship examination of The Royal College of Anaesthetists. This book consists of five complete sets of OSCE papers that closely simulate the OSCE format of the primary FRCA. To help both teachers and trainees in an objective assessment of their knowledge and skills, marks have been allocated to each OSCE. The tutorial following each OSCE station will provide a depth and breadth of knowledge for candidates and will assist trainers in setting up additional OSCEs on the related subject. Alongside the authors' previously published book *The Structured Oral Examination in Anaesthesia - Practice Papers for Teachers and Trainees* (ISBN 9780521680509), this book supplements the essential study material for the oral part of the primary FRCA examination.

The objective structured clinical examination is a valid tool for evaluating postgraduate clinical performance. We sincerely hope that the information in this book will be beneficial to trainees in their preparation for the FRCA examination and also for other equivalent postgraduate examinations and competency assessments. We wish you good luck with your revision and the exam.

Dr. Cyprian Mendonca MD FRCA
Consultant Anaesthetist
University Hospitals Coventry and Warwickshire
Coventry
UK

Dr. Shyam Balasubramanian MD FRCA
Consultant Anaesthetist
University Hospitals Coventry and Warwickshire
Coventry
UK

Foreword

Anaesthesia is not a career for the faint hearted. Progression through training requires passing the primary FRCA, accepted as being one of the most difficult postgraduate medical examinations. There are several hurdles: firstly, the MCQs, covering the three areas of physiology, pharmacology, and physics and clinical measurement; once successful, the lucky doctor has the challenge of tackling the structured oral examinations on the same day as the OSCEs.

Until recently, The Royal College of Anaesthetists was based in a beautiful, but relatively small building, in Russell Square. The burgeoning numbers of candidates could not be contained there for both parts of the exam. This resulted in added anxiety for the candidates, having to navigate around Bloomsbury to the various venues which accommodated the 'vivas', as they were known. Fortunately, the magnificent building now housing the College, in Red Lion Square, is able to host the whole exam.

The OSCEs instil terror in the minds of candidates. The sheer number of stations and brevity of each one demands a profound level of knowledge coupled with continual practice. This book is an invaluable aide to trainees sitting the exam. The stations are authentic, and the explanatory notes are so detailed that they are a valuable supplement to the standard textbooks. College tutors and other trainers will also find it helpful, not only as a source of revision, but also to assist them in setting up new practice stations.

The book is a perfect partner to the earlier published book, *The Structured Oral Examination in Anaesthesia - Practice Papers for Teachers and Trainees*; you will not be disappointed.

Jo James FRCA
Consultant Anaesthetist
Heart of England Foundation Trust &
Programme Director, Warwickshire School of Anaesthesia

Acknowledgements

We are grateful for the feedback and suggestions provided by trainees who attended the primary FRCA preparation courses at Coventry. Much of the material within has been used on the courses.

We are indebted to Dr. Jo James FRCA, Consultant Anaesthetist, Heart of England Foundation Trust and Programme Director, Warwickshire School of Anaesthesia, who critically reviewed the entire manuscript and made suggestions for the improvement of this book.

Our thanks are extended to Dr. Raja Lakshmanan FRCA, Specialist Registrar, Warwickshire School of Anaesthesia and Mr. Jason McAllister, Graphic Designer, University Hospitals Coventry and Warwickshire for their help with the illustrations, and also to Nikki Bramhill, Director, tfm publishing, for critically reviewing the manuscript.

We thank Dr. Jenny Layton-Henry, General Practitioner, Coventry, for her help with the case scenarios. We gratefully acknowledge the support and help received from our colleagues.

Abbreviations

ABG Arterial blood gas
Ach Acetylcholine
AF Atrial fibrillation
AIDS Acute immuno deficiency syndrome
ALS Advanced life support
AP Antero-posterior
APL Adjustable pressure limiting
APTT Activated partial thromboplastin time
ASA American Society of Anesthesiologists
AV Atrioventricular
BE Base excess
BiPAP Bi-level positive airway pressure
BURP Backward, upward and right-ward pressure
BW Bodyweight
CI Cardiac index
CICV Cannot intubate, cannot ventilate
CO Cardiac output
COAD Chronic obstructive airway disease
CPAP Continuous positive airway pressure
CPR Cardiopulmonary resuscitation
CRPS Complex regional pain syndrome
CSF Cerebrospinal fluid
CT Computer tomography
CVA Cerebrovascular accident
CVP Central venous pressure
DBS Double-burst stimulation
DC Direct current
DDAVP 1-Desamino-8-D arginine vasopressin
DIC Disseminated intravascular coagulation
DVT Deep vein thrombosis

ECG Electrocardiogram
ETT Endotracheal tube
FDP Fibrin degradation product
FEF Forced expiratory flow
FEV Forced expiratory volume
FFP Fresh frozen plasma
FGF Fresh gas flow
FRC Functional residual capacity
FVC Forced vital capacity
GA General anaesthesia
GCS Glasgow coma scale
GI Gastrointestinal
GP General practice
GT Greater trochanter
H/O History of
Hb Haemoglobin
Hct Haematocrit
HDU High dependency unit
HR Heart rate
ICP Intracranial pressure
ICU Intensive care unit
ID Internal diameter
IJV Internal jugular vein
INR International normalised ratio
IO Intra-osseous
IPPV Intermittent positive pressure ventilation
IV Intravenous
IVRA Intravenous regional anaesthesia
JVP Jugular venous pressure/pulse
LAD Left anterior descending
LBBB Left bundle branch block
LCA Left coronary artery
LED Light emitting diode
LFT Lacrimal, frontal and trochlear
LMA Laryngeal mask airway
MAC Minimum alveolar concentration
MAP Mean arterial pressure
MH Malignant hyperthermia

N Newton
NIBP Non-invasive blood pressure
NICE National Institute for Clinical Excellence
NSAID Non-steroidal anti-inflammatory drugs
OSAHS Obstructive sleep apnoea hypopnoea syndrome
PA Postero-anterior
Pa Pascal
PAP Pulmonary artery pressure
PAWP Pulmonary artery wedge pressure
PCA Patient controlled analgesia
PCI Percutaneous coronary intervention
PCW Pulmonary capillary wedge
PCWP Pulmonary capillary wedge pressure
PE Pulmonary embolism
PEA Pulseless electrical activity
PEEP Peak end expiratory pressure
PEFR Peak expiratory flow rate
PMH Past medical history
PONV Postoperative nausea and vomiting
PPM Parts per million
PSH Past surgical history
PSIS Posterior superior iliac spine
PSVT Paroxysmal supraventricular tachycardia
PT Prothrombin time
PTC Post-tetanic count
PVR Pulmonary vascular resistance
PVRI Pulmonary vascular resistance index
RA Right atrium
RBBB Right bundle branch block
RV Residual volume
RVH Right ventricular hypertrophy
SA Sino-atrial
SD Standard deviation
SI Systeme international
SVI Stroke volume index
SVR Systemic vascular resistance
SVRI Systemic vascular resistance index
SVT Supraventricular tachycardia

TLCO Transfer factor for carbon monoxide
TLC Total lung capacity
TOF Train of four
TRALI Transfusion-related acute lung injury
TTJV Transtracheal jet ventilation
VA Alveolar volume
VC Vital capacity
VF Ventricular fibrillation
VSD Ventricular septal defect
VT Ventricular tachycardia
WCC White cell count
WPW Wolff Parkinson White

OSCE
set 1

Station 1.1 Anaesthetic equipment: circle absorber

Information for the candidate

In this station you will be asked to check a breathing system as you routinely do before starting a list.

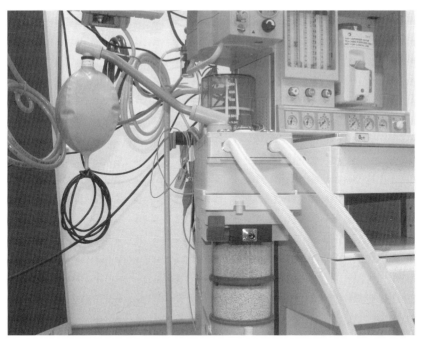

Figure 1.1a Anaesthetic machine with circle absorber system.

Examiner's mark sheet

Can you please check the breathing system on this anaesthetic machine?

marks

- ◆ Ensures that soda lime is present and is not used up (check colour).   1 ☐
- ◆ Visually inspects the system.   1 ☐
- ◆ Identifies the blocked filter.   2 ☐
- ◆ Appropriately performs the leak test.   2 ☐
- ◆ Identifies that it is leaking at the water drain.   2 ☐
- ◆ Checks function of the one-way valves by connecting bags at both ends.   2 ☐

What are the benefits in using this system?   4 ☐

- ◆ Economy: fresh gas flow (FGF) can be reduced to less than a litre per minute and consumption of volatile agents is reduced.
- ◆ Humidification: inspired gas will be saturated with water vapour from the expired gas.
- ◆ Reduced heat loss: in addition to conservation of heat, the exothermic reaction of CO_2 absorption assists in maintaining body temperature.
- ◆ Reduced atmospheric pollution: by using low FGF, escape of volatile anaesthetic agents into the atmosphere is minimised.

What happens if the unidirectional valve malfunctions?   1 ☐

Malfunction of the unidirectional valve leads to mixing of inspired gas with expired gas containing CO_2 and results in hypercapnla.

What is the mesh size of the granules?   1 ☐

4-8 mesh or 3-4mm spheres.

What do you understand by 4-8 mesh?   1 ☐

Strainers with 4 mesh have four equal strands per linear inch in both vertical and horizontal axes. Similarly, strainers with 8 mesh have 8 equal strands per linear inch in both vertical and horizontal axes. Granules of 4-8 mesh size pass through the strainers with 4-8 mesh.

What are the constituents of soda lime?   1 ☐

NaOH, $Ca(OH)_2$, KOH, water and silica.

Name some contaminants that can be produced in this system   2 ☐

Compound A and B are produced with sevoflurane. Desflurane, isofurane and enflurane react with dry soda lime to produce carbon monoxide. Methane and acetone are other compounds that may be produced.

Total:	/20

Information for the examiner

Ensure that the water drain is slightly opened to produce a leak. When you attach the filter, block the circuit with the plastic material from the package. The candidate should identify this during visual inspection or at the stage of performing the test for a leak.

Checking the circle system

This is one of the most commonly used breathing systems and the candidate should be thorough in their knowledge and skill related to this equipment.

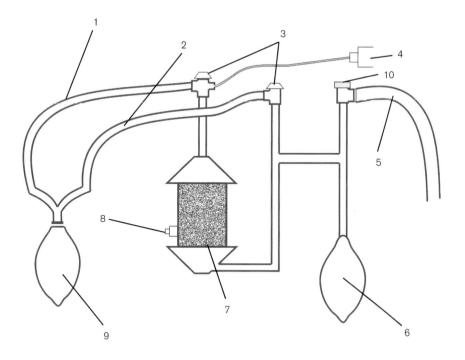

Figure 1.1b Components of the circle system.
1. Inspiratory limb; 2. Expiratory limb; 3. Unidirectional valve; 4. Fresh gas flow; 5. Scavenging; 6. Reservoir bag; 7. Soda lime canister; 8. Water drain; 9. Simulated lung; 10. APL valve.

Performing a leak check of a breathing system

- Set all gas flows to zero or minimum.
- Close the adjustable pressure limiting (APL) valve and occlude the Y-piece.
- Pressurise the breathing system to about 30cm H_2O with an oxygen flush.
- Ensure that pressure remains fixed for at least 10 seconds.
- Open the APL valve and ensure that pressure decreases.

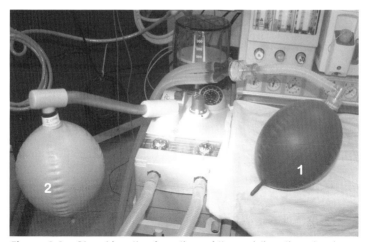

Figure 1.1c Checking the function of the unidirectional valves.
1. Simulated lung; 2. Reservoir bag.

Checking the unidirectional valve

- ◆ Place a second breathing bag (simulated lung) on the Y-piece.
- ◆ Fill the reservoir bag with an oxygen flush and manually ventilate.
- ◆ Ensure inflation and deflation of the simulated lung that is connected to the Y-piece; watch for movement of the unidirectional valves.

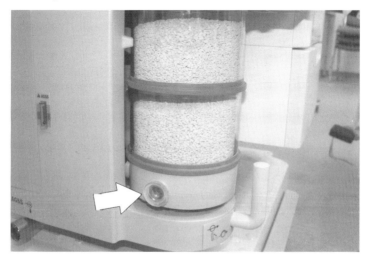

Figure 1.1d Water drain in the canister.

Chemical reactions during carbon dioxide absorption

First, CO_2 is dissolved in water to form carbonic acid, and then reacts with calcium hydroxide to form calcium carbonate and water. Carbon dioxide also reacts with sodium hydroxide to produce sodium bicarbonate, which then reacts with calcium hydroxide to regenerate sodium hydroxide.

◆ $CO_2 + H_2O \rightarrow H_2CO_3 \rightarrow H^+ + HCO_3^-$.

◆ $Ca(OH)_2 + H^+ + HCO_3^- \rightarrow CaCO_3 + 2H_2O$.

◆ $CO_2 + 2NaOH \rightarrow Na_2CO_3 + H_2O + heat$.

◆ $Na_2CO_3 + Ca(OH)_2 \rightarrow 2NaOH + CaCO_3$.

Water is required for the efficient absorption of CO_2. There is some moisture already present in the soda lime. More is added from the patient's expired gas and from the chemical reaction.

Functional analysis

During inspiration, fresh gas and the CO_2-free gas from the reservoir bag passes through the inspiratory unidirectional valve and inspiratory limb to the patient. During expiration, the inspiratory unidirectional valve closes and expired gas from the expiratory limb passes through the expiratory unidirectional valve to the soda lime canister.

Key points

◆ Visually inspect the system for integration, and continuity and completeness of the circuit.
◆ Verify that the canister is adequately filled with soda lime.
◆ Perform the leak test.
◆ Check the function of unidirectional valves.

Station 1.2 Data interpretation: ECG

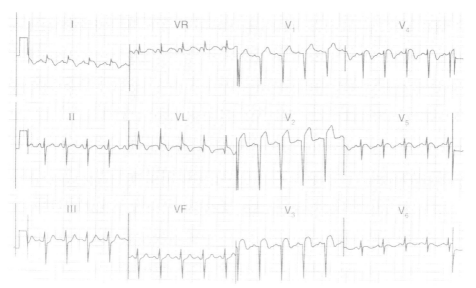

Figure 1.2a ECG 1.

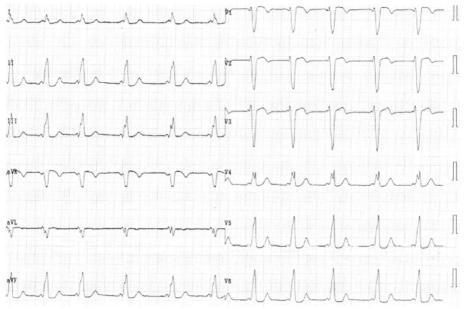

Figure 1.2b ECG 2.

Examiner's mark sheet

Please tick the correct answer - true or false.   *marks*

ECG 1

A 50-year-old male patient presented to the emergency department with chest pain of 6 hours duration. This is the ECG recorded at the time of admission.

1. Heart rate in this ECG is about 75 beats per minute.   True   False   2 ☐
2. This ECG is suggestive of an inferior infarction.   True   False   2 ☐
3. A blood test on admission is likely to show elevated troponin-T levels.   True   False   2 ☐
4. Aspirin should be given orally as soon as possible.   True   False   2 ☐
5. An angiogram would show occlusion of the left anterior descending (LAD) artery.   True   False   2 ☐

ECG 2

A 38-year-old female patient presented for micro-laryngeal surgery and has a history of paroxysmal palpitation. This is the ECG recorded during pre-operative assessment.

1. Standardisation in this ECG is 5mm = 1mV.   True   False   2 ☐
2. The PR interval is within normal limits.   True   False   2 ☐
3. Radiofrequency ablation is a treatment for this condition.   True   False   2 ☐
4. Digoxin is contra-indicated in this patient.   True   False   2 ☐
5. ECG shows left axis deviation.   True   False   2 ☐

Total: /20

Answers

ECG 1

1. False. The heart rate in this ECG is about 120 per minute. The ECG is recorded at a speed of 25mm per second; one large square on the ECG recording paper represents 0.20 sec and 300 large squares represent one minute. In the given ECG there are 2.5 large squares between two consecutive R waves. Since the rhythm is regular, the rate is calculated as 300/2.5 =120.

2. False. There is ST segment elevation in V1-V4, lead I and aVL suggesting an anterolateral infarction.

3. True. Although troponin-T peaks after 12 hours of myocardial infarction, it is detectable in serum about 3-6 hours after an acute myocardial infarction. Its level remains elevated for 14 days. Creatine kinase-MB (CK-MB) levels begin to rise within 4 hours after injury, peak at 18-24 hours, and return to normal over 3-4 days.

4. True. Aspirin in a dose of 150-300mg should be administered on diagnosing acute MI. Aspirin interferes with function of the enzyme cyclo-oxygenase and inhibits the formation of thromboxane A2. Aspirin prevents additional platelet activation, and interferes with platelet adhesion and cohesion.

5. True. The circumflex artery branch of the left coronary artery (LCA) and diagonal branches of the LAD are involved in an anterolateral infarct.

ECG 2

1. False. Standardisation is normal in this ECG; 10mm = 1mV.

2. False. It is 0.08 seconds in this ECG; reduced (Wolff-Parkinson-White [WPW] syndrome; see delta waves in II, III, aVF and V4-V6). The PR interval is measured from the beginning of the P wave to the beginning of the QRS complex. The normal interval is 0.12-0.2 seconds.

3. True. Radiofrequency ablation is the ideal treatment to destroy the abnormal pathway.

4. True. Digoxin, by slowing the normal atrioventricular (AV) conduction, facilitates conduction via an abnormal pathway.

5. False. QRS complexes are predominantly positive in both I and III. It is a normal axis.

The coronary arteries involved and ECG location in myocardial infarction are shown in Table 1.2.

Table 1.2 Coronary arteries involved and ECG location in myocardial infarction.

Wall affected	Leads showing ST elevation	Artery involved
Septal	V1, V2	LAD (septal perforators)
Anterior	V3, V4	LCA, LAD (diagonal branches)
Anteroseptal	V1, V2, V3, V4	LAD
Anterolateral	V3, V4, V5, V6, I, aVL	LAD, LCX, or obtuse marginal
Inferior	II, III, aVF	RCA or LCX
Lateral	I, aVL, V5, V6	LCX or obtuse marginal
Right ventricular (often associated with inferior)	II, III, aVF, V1, RV4, RV5	RCA

RCA = right coronary artery
LCA = left coronary artery
LAD = left anterior descending
LCX = circumflex

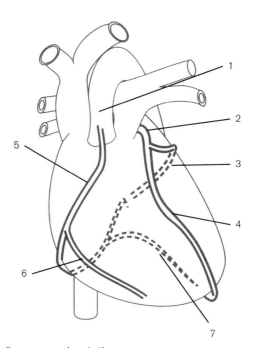

Figure 1.2c Coronary circulation.
1. Ascending aorta; 2. Left main coronary artery; 3. Circumflex artery; 4. Left anterior descending artery; 5. Right main coronary artery; 6. Marginal artery; 7. Posterior interventricular artery.

ECG 2 is suggestive of Wolff-Parkinson-White syndrome. In Wolff-Parkinson-White syndrome, an accessory pathway exists between the atria and ventricle, thereby causing early depolarisation of the ventricle. This results in a short PR interval and abnormal QRS complex on the ECG. A slurred upslope of the R wave is known as a delta (d) wave.

Key points

- Troponin-T has the greatest sensitivity and specificity in detecting acute myocardial infarction. It is normally not found in the serum and is released only when myocardial necrosis occurs.
- Aspirin has been shown to decrease mortality and reinfarction rates after myocardial infarction. Clopidogrel is an alternative choice in patients with an aspirin allergy.
- Recent evidence suggests that primary percutaneous coronary intervention (PCI) is more effective than thrombolysis.

Station 1.3 Data interpretation: haemodynamic data

Information for the candidate

A 39-year-old lady was admitted to intensive care from a medical ward where she was treated for pneumonia and diabetes mellitus. She is intubated and ventilated. Two hours following intensive treatment the following parameters were observed.

◆ HR: 126/minute, BP: 80 /42 (54) mmHg, CVP: +4 mmHg.

◆ Blood glucose: 24mmol/L; temperature: 38.2°C; Hb: 10gm/dl; WCC: 18.5 x 10^9L.

◆ pH: 7.16; PCO_2: 5.85kPa; PaO_2: 15.7kPa (FiO_2 of 0.8, PEEP of 8cmH_2O).

◆ HCO_3^-: 14mmol/L; BE: -16mmol/L; lactate 3.2mmol/L.

◆ Body surface area: 2m^2; cardiac-output: 8L/min; stroke volume: 80ml.

◆ PA pressure: 25/7(13) mmHg; PAWP: 6 mmHg; SvO_2: 65%; CaO_2: 15ml/dl.

Examiner's mark sheet

Please tick the correct answer - true or false.   *marks*

1. Cardiac index is 4L/m^2.   True False 2 ☐
2. Stroke index is 40ml/m^2.   True False 2 ☐
3. Systemic vascular resistance would be   True False 2 ☐
   500dyn.s.cm^{-5}.
4. This patient needs more intravenous fluids.   True False 2 ☐
5. This patient needs a norepinephrine infusion.   True False 2 ☐
6. Oxygen delivery (DO_2) would be 120ml/minute.   True False 2 ☐
7. This patient has a high oxygen extraction ratio.   True False 2 ☐

8. Intravenous sodium bicarbonate is the treatment of choice.   True False 2 ☐

9. Haemodynamic data are suggestive of cardiogenic shock.   True False 2 ☐

10. This patient needs a blood transfusion to increase DO_2.   True False 2 ☐

Total: /20

Answers

1. True. The cardiac index is cardiac output (CO) per body surface area, $8L/2m^2 = 4L/m^2$.

2. True. Stroke volume/body surface area, $80ml/2m^2 = 40ml/m^2$.

3. True. SVR: (MAP - CVP/CO) x 80; (54 - 4/8) x 80; (50/8) x 80 = $500dyn.s.cm^{-5}$.

4. True.This patient is hypotensive, has a low central venous pressure (CVP) and low wedge pressure.

5. True. This patient has a low systemic vascular resistance (SVR).

6. False. Oxygen delivery = CaO_2 (ml/dl) x 10 x CO (L) = 15 x 8 x 10 =1200ml/min.

7. True. Oxygen delivery is 1200ml/minute and mixed venous saturation is low (65%), suggesting increased oxygen extraction.

8. False. In this patient the cause of acidosis is most likely due to inadequate tissue perfusion. The primary aim is to improve tissue perfusion.

9. False. This patient has a high CO, low CVP and low pulmonary artery wedge pressure (PAWP).

10. False. Blood transfusion is not indicated at a haemoglobin of 10gm/dl.

Normal haemodynamic values

Cardiac index (CI): $2.8\text{-}3.5\text{L/min/m}^2$.
SVR: $900\text{-}1200\ \text{dynes.s.cm}^{-5}$.
SVRI: $1700\text{-}2600\ \text{dynes.s.cm}^{-5}.\text{m}^2$.
PVR: $120\text{-}200\ \text{dynes.s.cm}^{-5}$.
PVRI: $210\text{-}360\ \text{dynes.s.cm}^{-5}.\text{m}^2$.
O_2 extraction ratio: 0.22-0.33.
O_2 consumption index: $100\text{-}180\text{ml/min/m}^2$.
O_2 delivery index: $520\text{-}720\text{ml/min/m}^2$.

Haemodynamic calculations

SVR: (MAP-CVP/CO) x 80.
PVR: (PAP-PAWP/CO) x 80.
SVRI: (MAP-CVP/CI) x 80.
PVRI: (PAP-PAWP/CI) x 80.

DO_2: CO x CaO_2 x 10.
CaO_2: Hb x SaO_2 x 1.34/100.
Oxygen extraction ratio: CaO_2 - CvO_2 / CaO_2.

Septic shock

Common sources of sepsis include the abdomen, chest, urinary tract, wounds, and intravascular lines. The presence of severe infection triggers a massive systemic inflammatory response with systemic activation of leucocytes and release of a variety of potentially damaging mediators. These mediators cause profound vasodilatation, increased capillary permeability and myocardial depression. The microvascular changes include increased permeability, micro-embolisation and arteriovenous shunting.

The oxygen extraction ratio = VO_2/DO_2. An increase in the oxygen extraction ratio results in a decrease in mixed venous oxygen saturation and vice versa. Normal mixed venous oxygen saturation is 70-75%. Depending upon the stage of sepsis the oxygen extraction can increase (as in hypermetabolic states) or decrease (when cellular metabolism is disturbed and cells are unable to use oxygen).

Key points

- A systemic inflammatory response and sepsis causes profound vasodilatation and a low systemic vascular resistance.
- Inadequate tissue perfusion results in metabolic acidosis.
- pH indicates a primary acid base disorder.
- The metabolic component of the acid base disorder is indicated by the level of bicarbonate in the plasma.

Station 1.4 Data interpretation: statistics

Information for the candidate

In this station you will be shown a correlation-regression graph and will be questioned on statistics.

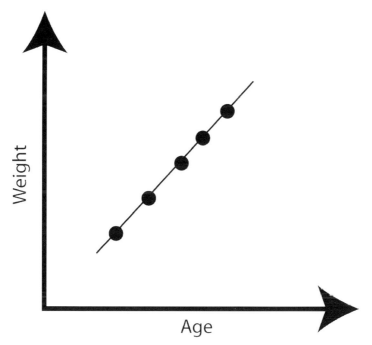

Figure 1.4 Correlation-regression graph: age and weight of children.

Examiner's mark sheet

Please tick the correct answer - true or false.   *marks*

1. The graph illustrates a positive correlation.   True False 2 ☐
2. The correlation coefficient is denoted by the letter 'r'. True False 2 ☐
3. It is customary to plot the dependent variable along   True False 2 ☐
    the horizontal x-axis.
4. It is possible to have a correlation coefficient of 1.1. True False 2 ☐
5. It is possible to have a correlation coefficient of -0.7. True False 2 ☐
6. The correlation coefficient of 0.7 is statistically   True False 2 ☐
    significant.
7. Regression involves estimating the best straight   True False 2 ☐
    line to summarise the association.
8. A complete absence of correlation is represented   True False 2 ☐
    by 0.
9. Correlation implies causation.   True False 2 ☐
10. These data could be analysed using a non-   True False 2 ☐
    parametric test.

Total: /20

Answers

1. True. Weight increases as age increases, thus a positive correlation.

2. True.

3. False. Here, age is the independent variable and is plotted on the x-axis.

4. False.

5. True. r ranges from +1 to -1.

6. True. 0.7 signifies a strong association.

7. True.

8. True.

9. False.

10. True.

Key points

◆ A correlation denotes an association between two quantitative variables.
◆ Regression involves estimating the best straight line to summarise the association.
◆ The correlation coefficient (r) measures the degree of association and is measured on a scale that varies from +1 through 0 to -1.
◆ When one variable increases as the other increases, the correlation is positive; when one decreases as the other increases, the correlation is negative.
◆ Complete absence of correlation is represented by 0.
◆ The independent variable, such as time or age, is measured along the x-axis.
◆ Correlation is not causation.
◆ The strength of association for absolute values of r: 0-0.19 is very weak; 0.2-0.39 is weak; 0.4-0.59 is moderate; 0.6-0.79 is strong; 0.8-1 is very strong.
◆ The significance of data can be tested using a t-test for parametric data or a non-parametric test, such as a Spearman rank correlation.

Station 1.5 Anatomy: internal jugular vein

Information for the candidate

This station is for the purpose of exploring knowledge on anatomy of the internal jugular vein and its cannulation.

Examiner's mark sheet

marks

Describe the course of the internal jugular vein (IJV)   2 ☐

The IJV originates at the jugular foramen (continues with the sigmoid sinus) and runs down the neck, to terminate behind the sternoclavicular joint, where it joins the subclavian vein to form the brachiocephalic vein.

State the relations of the IJV   3 ☐

- Anterior: internal carotid artery and vagus nerve. The sternocleidomastoid muscle is in the lower part and the vagus lies between the vein and artery.
- Posterior: sympathetic chain and the dome of the pleura. On the left side, the IJV lies anterior to the thoracic duct.
- Medial: carotid arteries and cranial nerves IX-XII. The deep cervical lymph nodes lie close to the vein.

Name the tributaries that drain into the IJV   3 ☐

Common facial vein, lingual vein, superior and middle thyroid veins and pharyngeal venous plexus.

Demonstrate the insertion of this central line via the IJV   8 ☐
(on the manikin)

- Sterile technique; 15°-20° head down tilt.
- Local anaesthetic infiltration to skin.
- Describes the use of ultrasound.
- Appropriate site of skin puncture and correct direction of needle.
- Aspiration of blood and insertion of guidewire.
- Passes the dilator and then railroads the CVP catheter over the guidewire.
- Aspirates all lumens and sutures the line in place.
- Obtains a chest X-ray.

What are the complications of central line placement?   4 ☐

Complications can be categorised as mechanical, infective and thrombotic.

Mechanical complications occur either due to needling or secondary to the introduction and presence of the catheter. They include haemorrhage, pneumothorax, haemothorax, air embolism, nerve damage, extravascular catheter placement and chylothorax.

Total:	/20

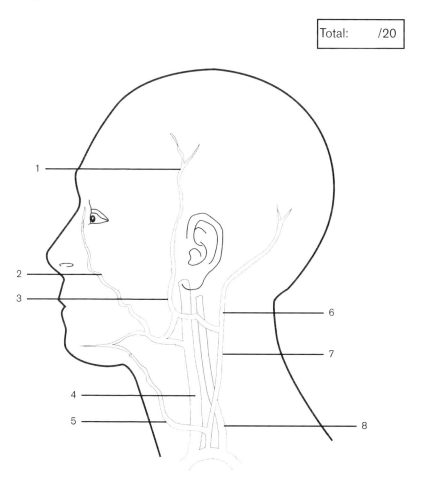

Figure 1.5a Veins of the head and neck.
1. Superficial temporal vein; 2. Facial vein; 3. Retromandibular vein; 4. Internal jugular vein; 5. Anterior jugular vein; 6. Posterior auricular vein; 7. External jugular vein; 8. Vertebral vein.

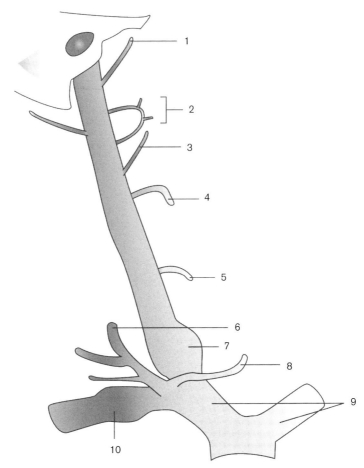

Figure 1.5b Tributaries of the IJV
1. Inferior petrosal vein; 2. Pharyngeal veins; 3. Facial vein; 4. Superior thyroid vein; 5. Middle thyroid vein; 6. External jugular vein; 7. Internal jugular vein; 8. Anterior jugular vein; 9. Brachiocephalic veins; 10. Subclavian vein.

Major veins of the head and neck

The IJV is the continuation of the sigmoid sinus. It runs down the side of the neck in a vertical direction, lying, at first, lateral to the internal carotid artery, and then lateral to the common carotid artery. The glossopharyngeal and hypoglossal nerves pass forward between the IJV and internal carotid artery. The vagus nerve descends between and behind the vein and artery in the same sheath.

The IJV receives many tributaries within the neck. During its course it receives the inferior petrosal sinus, common facial, lingual, pharyngeal, superior and middle thyroid veins, and sometimes the occipital vein.

The external jugular vein commences in the substance of the parotid gland at the level of the mandible. It passes downwards to the midpoint of the clavicle and enters the subclavian vein. In its course it crosses the sternocleidomastoid muscle.

Key points

- The right internal jugular vein has a straighter course and is more commonly used for cannulation.
- NICE recommends the use of 2-D ultrasound guidance in order to reduce associated complications.
- The steps involved in central venous cannulation include preparation of the patient (assessing indication/contra-indication, explanation of procedure, consent), preparation of the site (positioning, aseptic precautions) and then the actual technique. Confirm the position of the catheter with X-ray.
- Complications involved with central venous cannulation can be mechanical, infective or thrombotic. They can be immediate or delayed.

Station 1.6 Communication: awake tracheal intubation

Information for the candidate

A 70-year-old male patient is scheduled for an elective laparoscopic cholecystectomy. His previous anaesthetic history is: failed intubation for an umbilical hernia repair; grade 4 (Cormack and Lehane) laryngoscopic view; and bag and mask ventilation was easy. The patient was woken up from general anaesthesia and surgery was performed under spinal anaesthesia.

Explain to the patient about awake fibreoptic intubation for his laparoscopic cholecystectomy.

Examiner's mark sheet

marks

Introduces him/herself to the patient.   1 ☐

Asks about the patient's understanding regarding his previous   1 ☐
anaesthetic problem.

Explains the need for intubation (breathing tube).   2 ☐

Explains how it is normally done.   1 ☐

Explains why it needs to be done differently this time.   2 ☐

Other alternative methods are available (fibreoptic intubation   1 ☐
after induction of GA).

Able to explain the disadvantages of fibreoptic intubation after   2 ☐
induction of GA (there is a possibility of failure to intubate
which is unsafe and further danger may arise due to the
possible difficulty in ventilation using a bag and mask).

Explains the benefits of awake fibreoptic intubation (an awake   2 ☐
patient is able to maintain the airway, which is safer than any
other alternative method).

Explains about sedation during the procedure.   2 ☐

Explains about adequate monitoring.   1 ☐

Gives a satisfactory explanation of local anaesthetic   2 ☐
technique.

Compares the technique with endoscopy or something else familiar to the patient.   1 ☐

Uses simple terms (telescope or camera).   1 ☐

Overall clarity of communication and an ability to establish rapport with the patient.   1 ☐

Total:	/20

Information for the actor

There was difficulty in inserting the breathing tube into your windpipe during your last anaesthetic. The anaesthetist had to wake you up. The surgery was done with an injection in the back, uneventfully. Your previous anaesthetist advised you to warn subsequent anaesthetists about the problem. The anaesthetist this time is planning to insert the breathing tube into your windpipe while you are awake. Understandably, you are scared and anxious. You are concerned that it may be very painful to pass the tube.

Awake fibreoptic intubation

Awake fibreoptic intubation is indicated in known or suspected difficult intubation, when there is an aspiration risk and difficult intubation is anticipated, and when there is known or suspected cervical cord instability.

Relative contra-indications include upper airway bleeding or a bleeding tendency, stridor and unco-operative patients.

The patient should be fully monitored during the procedure, an intravenous access should be secured and supplementary oxygen should be administered via a nasal catheter or through a fibreoptic scope. Judicious sedation may be required. Naloxone and flumazenil should be available.

The technique can be performed either from the conventional position from the head end with the patient supine or, in a sitting up, semi-reclined position with the operator standing in front.

The nasal route has the advantage of a better anatomical alignment with the vocal cords. But passing the tube through nostrils in an awake patient can be uncomfortable.

Techniques of airway anaesthesia

There is a wide range of options available to anaesthetise the airway for awake intubation.

Anaesthesia to the nasal passage and nasopharynx with a cocaine solution or paste is commonly used. Cocaine is also a vasoconstrictor. The total recommended dose is 1.5mg/Kg. Lidocaine 5% with 0.5% phenylephrine is a suitable alternative.

Anaesthesia for the oropharynx with lidocaine 4% solution is suitable for oral analgesia. The patient is asked to gargle 4-5ml of solution. This can be supplemented with 3 to 4 sprays of 10% lidocaine (each spray contains 10mg of lidocaine). Lidocaine 2% gel is a suitable alternative for providing analgesia to the tongue and oropharynx.

Nebulisation of local anaesthetic (4% lidocaine) is a simple technique and provides partial analgesia to both the upper and lower airway. Larger particles settle in the upper airway, smaller particles reach the lower airway. This technique is useful, particularly if coughing needs to be minimised.

The lower airway can be anaesthetised using topical anaesthesia or with nerve blocks, topical anaesthesia being more popular.

In the spray as you go technique, 4% lidocaine is injected via the working channel of the fibreoptic scope. An epidural catheter is passed down the working channel of the scope; this allows direct visualisation and application of local anaesthetic solution close to the anatomical structures to be anaesthetised. Following topical anaesthesia to the nasal passage and oropharynx, the fibreoptic scope is advanced until the base of the tongue and epiglottis is seen. 1-2ml of 4% lidocaine should be sprayed onto the base of the tongue and epiglottis. Another 1-2ml of local anaesthetic is sprayed onto the glottis and vocal cords. Then the fibreoptic scope is advanced further close to the glottis and an additional 1ml of local anaesthetic is sprayed through the vocal cords into the trachea. A total of

3-6ml of 4% lidocaine may be required. This technique will provide satisfactory anaesthesia for awake fibreoptic intubation.

The internal laryngeal nerve (branch of the superior laryngeal nerve) can be blocked either by an internal or external approach. The hyoid bone is located directly above the thyroid cartilage. The greater horn is located in the lateral most part of the hyoid bone. The superior laryngeal nerve can be blocked by walking a 25G needle inferiorly off the greater horn and injecting 2ml of 2% lidocaine. Accidental arterial injection (into the carotid) is a possible complication.

The internal laryngeal nerve runs just under the mucous membrane covering the pyriform fossa, where it can be easily blocked by applying a cotton wool ball soaked in 2% lidocaine, using Krause's forceps. The oropharynx and the posterior two thirds of the tongue need to be anaesthetised before performing this block.

In translaryngeal anaesthesia, the skin over the cricothyroid membrane is infiltrated with local anaesthetic. Then a needle or cannula attached to a syringe containing normal saline is inserted through the cricothyroid membrane; the needle should be directed backwards and caudad to avoid trauma to the vocal cords. Correct placement is confirmed by aspiration of air via the needle. 2-4ml of 4% lidocaine should be injected at the end of inspiration. During the process the patient coughs and anaesthesia should spread both above and below the cords.

Topical anaesthesia to the nasal cavity and oropharynx, followed by transbronchoscopic administration of lidocaine is more straightforward and often tolerated by patients.

Key points

- Antisialogogues are used to reduce secretion and improve the endoscopic view.
- Skilled assistance is mandatory during the procedure.
- The patient should fully understand the need for the procedure
- Awake intubation is a safe way of securing the airway.
- Reassure the patient that the procedure as such is not painful.
- The patient is likely to cough while anaesthetising the larynx and trachea.
- The patient's co-operation for a local anaesthetic technique is vital.

Station 1.7 Technical skill: cricothyrotomy

Information for the candidate

A 20-year-old patient presented for appendicectomy. Rapid sequence induction of general anesthesia was attempted. Laryngoscopy revealed a grade 4 view, and the bag and mask ventilation failed. The patient is desaturating to 80%. A 'cannot intubate, cannot ventilate' (CICV) scenario has arisen and it is decided to resort to emergency cricothyrotomy and transtracheal jet ventilation (TTJV).

Examiner's mark sheet

marks

Can you perform cricothyrotomy on this manikin?   1 ☐

◆ Preparation: checks the equipment.

What equipment do you need for TTJV?   2 ☐

Intravenous (venflon) type cannula, i.e. over the needle catheter (14G) or a jet ventilation catheter (13G), a syringe filled with saline, a manual jet ventilation device or a Sanders injector.

Proceed with the cricothyrotomy

◆ Uses aseptic technique.   1 ☐
◆ Palpates the landmarks: thyroid cartilage, cricoid   3 ☐
cartilage, cricothyroid membrane.
◆ Stabilises the cricoid with thumb and middle finger.   1 ☐
◆ Puncture site: midline.   1 ☐
◆ Directs the needle at a 45° angle caudally.   1 ☐
◆ Aspirates air.   1 ☐
◆ Advances the catheter or cannula and removes the needle.   1 ☐
◆ Aspirates again to check the cannula is in place.   1 ☐
◆ Connects the jet and ventilates (press the lever for 1 to 2   1 ☐
seconds).

Why choose the cricothyroid membrane? 2

It is superficial and is relatively avascular. The cricoid cartilage is a complete ring and, therefore, holds the airway open.

Give two complications of cricothyrotomy 2 ☐

- ◆ Bleeding.
- ◆ Oesophageal perforation.
- ◆ Posterior tracheal wall perforation.
- ◆ Surgical emphysema.
- ◆ Barotrauma (pneumothorax).

Describe two precautions you would take to prevent 2 ☐
barotrauma

After first inflation, make sure that the chest is deflating. If there is a complete airway obstruction, insert a second cannula for expiration.

Total:	/20

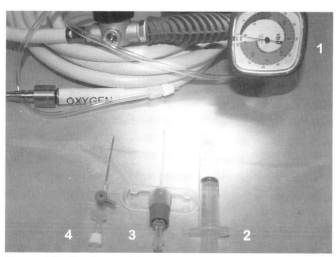

Figure 1.7a Equipment for emergency cricothyrotomy.
1. Manual jet ventilator (Manujet III); 2. Saline filled syringe; 3. 13G jet ventilation catheter; 4. 14G cannula.

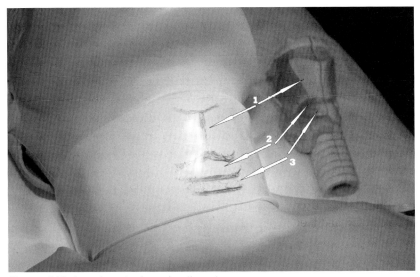

Figure 1.7b Landmarks for cricothyrotomy.
1. Thyroid cartilage; 2. Cricothyroid membrane; 3. Cricoid cartilage.

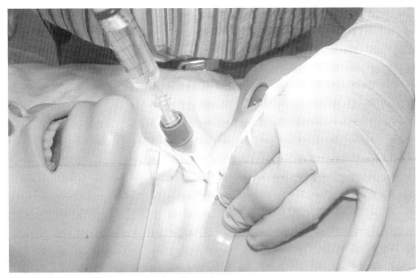

Figure 1.7c Technique of cricothyrotomy.

Emergency cricothyrotomy

The cricothyroid membrane is subcutaneous in the midline and is located between the strap muscles of the neck. It is on average 8mm deep below the skin (the range is 3-14mm). In adults it is 9mm high and 22-30mm wide, but the width between cricothyroid muscles is about 9mm. Therefore, the largest tube that can be passed should have an outer diameter of less than 9mm (a 6mm tracheostomy tube has an outer diameter of 8.3mm). A 6mm size cuffed tracheostomy tube is commonly used.

For identifying the cricoid cartilage use the index finger to identify the thyroid notch and then follow the finger downwards in the midline. A dip is felt below the thyroid cartilage; this is the cricothyroid space. A prominent structure felt immediately below this is the cricoid cartilage. Once identified, stabilise the cricoid cartilage with the thumb and middle finger, and using the index finger locate the cricothyroid membrane in the midline. If the thyroid cartilage is not prominent, then palpate the trachea at the suprasternal notch, grasp between the thumb and middle finger, and follow the index finger upwards to palpate the cricothyroid membrane.

Emergency cricothyrotomy is performed in a 'cannot intubate, cannot ventilate' scenario to oxygenate the patient.

The following are the three different techniques for emergency cricothyrotomy.

1. In needle cricothyrotomy and transtracheal jet ventilation, a 13G cricothyrotomy cannula or a 14G venflon is commonly used. The small cannula has a high resistance and needs a high pressure oxygen source to ventilate. A jet injector at 1-4 bar pressure (Sanders injector or Manujet injector) is used. Exhalation is passive and must occur through the pharynx and larynx. In the case of complete airway obstruction, a second cannula through the cricothyroid membrane may be required to facilitate exhalation.

2. A large purpose-made cannula with an internal diameter of 4mm or more allows ventilation of the lungs using an anaesthetic breathing system.

3. Surgical cricothyrotomy with a rapid four-step technique involves:

- Palpation of the cricothyroid membrane.
- A horizontal stab incision over the cricothyroid space.
- Traction with a tracheal hook. A scalpel handle inserted through the skin incision is then rotated 90°.
- Downward traction with a tracheal hook and intubation with a tracheostomy tube.

Key points

- Locate the cricoid cartilage.
- The cricothyroid membrane should be punctured in the midline.
- After the first inflation, ensure that the chest is deflating before further inflations, to avoid the risk of barotrauma.

Station 1.8 Clinical examination: assessment of a trauma patient

Information for the candidate

You are called to Accident and Emergency to see a middle-aged male patient who has been involved in a road traffic accident. You have a single assistant, an experienced paramedic. The rest of the trauma team are on their way and will arrive in 5 minutes.

Examiner's mark sheet

marks

The patient has a head injury

Controls cervical spine throughout.   2 ☐
A - Assesses airway.   1 ☐
States low conscious level will require definitive airway (here   1 ☐
or at D).

B - Assesses breathing.   1 ☐
C - Attaches monitoring.   1 ☐
Asks for cardiovascular parameters or assesses them (BP: 2 ☐
130/70 mmHg, HR: 74 bpm, capillary refill: 2 seconds).

The airway is clear; breath sounds are normal and the patient is haemodynamically stable

Establishes intravenous access.   1 ☐
D - Assesses Glasgow coma scale (GCS).   3 ☐
Assesses pupils.   1 ☐

Examination of the pupils shows one side to be fixed and dilated. GCS is 13; eyes: open to verbal commands = 3, movement on command = 6, vocal: confused = 4

What radiological investigations would you request in a trauma scenario?   2 ☐

X-rays of neck (c-spine), chest and pelvis.

What is the definitive care plan for this head-injury patient?   2 ☐

CT scan and a neurosurgical opinion/referral.

How would you transfer this patient to have a CT scan?   2 ☐

Make sure that the patient is stable; ensure that the patient's airway is protected, otherwise the airway needs to be secured with tracheal intubation. Ensure that venous access is secured, monitoring is established and emergency drugs are available.

The CT scan shows an extradural haematoma. What is the treatment?   1 ☐

Transfer to the neurosurgical unit and evacuation of the haematoma.

Total:	/20

Information for the actor

You will be playing the role of a patient who was involved in a road traffic accident and sustained a head injury.

A doctor will be assessing your injuries to plan appropriate treatment. You have to lie still on a couch when the doctor examines you, open your eyes to command and move your legs or arms only when he asks you to do so. If he/she asks you to squeeze his/her finger then you can respond. If he/she asks any questions you can give some inappropriate answers to show them that you are confused.

Assessment of a trauma patient

Management of a trauma patient involves a rapid primary survey, resuscitation of vital functions, more detailed secondary assessment and initiation of definitive care. In this OSCE, during the given 5 minutes of time, the candidate should demonstrate knowledge and skill of a primary survey. The cervical spine should be initially immobilised by manual inline traction and later immobilised using a semi-rigid collar and two bolsters on either side of the head and neck strapped to the spine board.

To identify life-threatening injuries during a primary survey, the ABCDE (airway, breathing, circulation, disability and exposure) sequence should be followed.

Indications for a CT scan in a head injury patient

- GCS 12/15 or less.
- Confusion or drowsiness (GCS 13 or 14/15), followed by failure to improve within at most 4 hours of clinical observation.
- GCS 15/15 - but with severe nausea and vomiting, severe persistent headache, irritability and altered behaviour or seizure.
- Deteriorating level of consciousness.
- Progressive focal neurological signs.
- New focal neurological signs.

Indications for a neurosurgical referral

- Persisting coma (GCS score 8/15 or less) after initial resuscitation.
- Confusion which persists for more than 4 hours.
- Deterioration in level of consciousness after admission (a sustained drop of one point on the motor or verbal subscales, or two points on the eye opening subscale of the GCS).
- Progressive focal neurological signs.
- A seizure without full recovery.
- Compound depressed skull fracture.
- Definite or suspected penetrating injury.
- A cerebrospinal fluid (CSF) leak or other sign of a basal fracture.

Key points

- The ABCDE sequence should be followed during a primary survey to identify and manage life-threatening injuries.
- Protecting the cervical spine is most important during airway assessment and management.
- During a secondary survey a complete neurological examination should be performed, including the GCS score.

Station 1.9 Measuring equipment: pulmonary artery flotation catheter

Information for the candidate

In this station you will be asked questions about invasive cardiac monitoring.

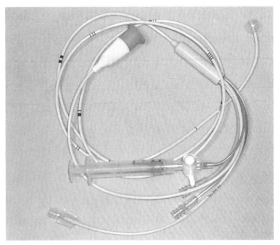

Figure 1.9a.

Examiner's mark sheet

marks

Can you identify this?   1 ☐

Pulmonary artery flotation catheter.

What is the normal pulmonary capillary wedge   1 ☐
pressure?

4-12 mmHg.

Where will the proximal lumen open? How far is it from 2 ☐
the tip and what does it measure?

Into the right atrium; 25cm from the tip; it measures CVP.

What is the volume of the balloon in the tip?   1 ☐

Approximately 1.5ml.

Can you draw the various traces as the pulmonary artery flotation catheter is inserted and wedged? 4 ☐

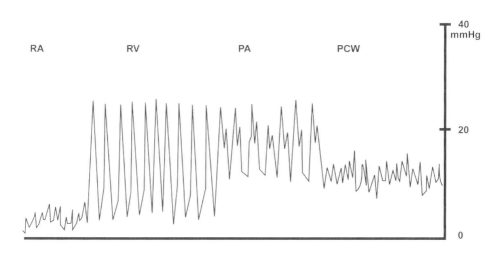

Figure 1.9b Pulmonary artery catheter trace.
RA: right atrium, RV: right ventricle, PA: pulmonary artery, PCW: pulmonary capillary wedge.

What will the trace resemble if the catheter coils back into the right atrium? 1 ☐

It will resemble the trace of the CVP.

Where is the thermistor situated in the catheter? 1 ☐

4cm proximal to the tip of the catheter.

State at least two uses of this catheter 2 ☐

◆ Assessment of volume status where the CVP is unreliable.

- Sampling of mixed venous blood to calculate shunt fraction.
- Measurement of cardiac output using thermodilution.
- Derivation of other cardiovascular indices, such as the pulmonary vascular resistance (PVR), oxygen delivery and uptake.

State at least three complications of using this catheter

3

- Arrhythmias on insertion.
- Knotting of the catheter in the right ventricle.
- Balloon rupture.
- Pulmonary infarction.

State at least two measured values and two derived haemodynamic variables obtained from a pulmonary artery catheter

2+2

- Measured values: CVP, PAP, PCWP, CO, SVO_2.
- Derived variables: cardiac index, stroke volume, SVI, SVR, SVRI, PVR, PVRI.

Total:	/20

Key points

- The pulmonary artery flotation catheter was first described by Swan and Ganz in 1970. It is 7 or 7.5 FG in size and 110cm long.
- There is a balloon at the tip which has a capacity of 1.5ml.
- A thermistor is located about 4cm proximal to the tip.
- Before inserting the catheter, it should be connected to the transducer, which should be zeroed. By gently waving the catheter up and down, the corresponding wave should appear on the monitor, ensuring that the catheter is connected to the correct transducer.

- The catheter should then be advanced 20cm before inflating the balloon.
- Whilst the catheter is in the right atrium, the CVP waveform is displayed on the monitor. When the catheter enters the right ventricle this waveform changes with a systolic pressure of 25 mmHg and diastolic pressure of 0-5 mmHg. The waveform suddenly changes as the catheter enters the pulmonary artery. Systolic pressure in the pulmonary artery is the same as that of the right ventricle, but diastolic pressure is higher (10-12 mmHg).
- As the catheter advances through the pulmonary artery it will eventually wedge in a small branch and PAWP is displayed, which reflects the left ventricular filling pressure.

Station 1.10 Resuscitation: paediatric resuscitation

Information for the candidate

A 5-year-old child has collapsed on the ward. There is no nurse available and you are on your own.

Examiner's mark sheet

marks

SAFE approach (1 x 5)   5 ☐

1. Checks responsiveness and requests help.
2. Opens the airway and a chin lift and jaw thrust is performed.
3. Assesses the airway by look, listen, feel.
4. Five rescue breaths are given, if not breathing.
5. Checks the pulse (carotid pulse for 10 seconds).

6. Starts CPR at 15 chest compressions: two rescue   2 ☐
   breaths (correct method of chest compression).

How many compressions per minute?   1 ☐

100/minute.

When would you call for a resuscitation team?   1 ☐

After 1 minute of CPR.

Now the help arrives and the monitor shows this rhythm

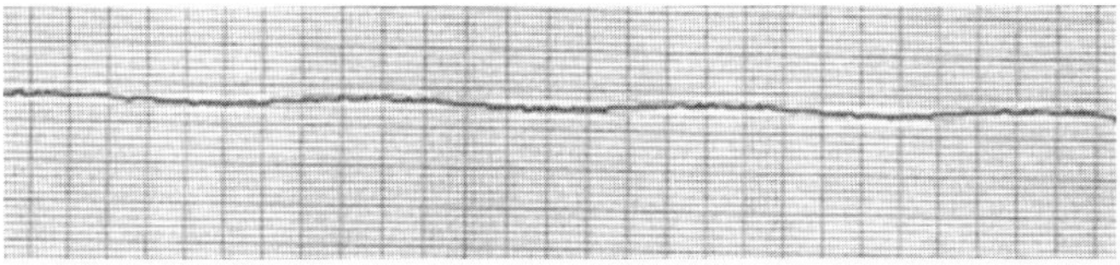

Figure 1.10 ECG.

What is the management?   4 ☐

Immediately resume CPR 15:2 for 2 minutes.

During CPR:

- Corrects reversible causes.
- Checks electrode position and contact.
- Attempts/verifies: IV/IO access; airway and oxygen.
- Gives uninterrupted compressions when the trachea is intubated.
- Gives adrenaline every 3-5 minutes.
- Considers atropine.

What is the initial intravenous (IV) dose of adrenaline?   2 ☐

10µg/Kg (0.1ml/Kg of 1: 10 000 adrenaline).

What is the intra-osseous dose of adrenaline?   1 ☐

10µg/Kg.

How much would you give through the tracheal tube?   1   ☐

100µg/Kg.

What will be the approximate weight of this child?   2   ☐

18Kg (2 x [age+4]).

What is the volume of IV fluid you would administer to   1   ☐
this child as an initial bolus?

360ml (20ml/Kg).

Total:	/20

Paediatric life support

After ensuring the safety of both rescuer and child, check the responsiveness, followed by airway and breathing. If the child is not breathing or is making agonal gasps, deliver five rescue breaths followed by one minute CPR before calling for a resuscitation team.

With chest compression, the ventilation ratio for children of all ages is 15:2 (lay rescuers are taught to use 30:2 ratio). In infants, a two-finger compression technique is used when there is only one rescuer. If there are two or more rescuers, then the chest can be compressed using the two-thumb encircling technique. In older children the lower third of the sternum should be compressed with the heel of one hand. The sternum should be compressed one fingerbreadth above the xiphisternum. The compression should be sufficient to depress the sternum by one third of the depth of the chest. The chest compression should be continued uninterruptedly when the trachea is intubated.

Vascular access can be difficult in small children and if there is no success after three attempts, an intra-osseous (IO) needle should be inserted. The onset of drug action and the time to achieve plasma concentration are similar to those provided by a central venous route. Fluid resuscitation using 20ml/Kg of isotonic crystalloid is indicated for volume expansion. It can be repeated after reassessing. The recommended dose of intravenous or intra-osseous adrenaline is 10µg/Kg and can be repeated every 3-5 minutes during CPR. Ventricular fibrillation or pulseless ventricular tachycardia should be treated with prompt defibrillation. The recommended energy is 4J/Kg for all shocks (monophasic or biphasic defibrillators).

Key points

- Ensure the safety of rescuer and child.
- Open the airway by a chin lift, and, if required, use a jaw thrust. A gentle head tilt can be performed if a cervical spine injury is not suspected. Do not take more than 10 seconds to assess the breathing.
- Soon after recognising abnormal or absent breathing, give 5 rescue breaths followed by one minute of CPR, then call for a resuscitation team.
- Administer high flow oxygen.
- For chest compression (in children >1 years of age), the sternum should be compressed by approximately one third the depth of the chest.

(For further reading please refer to the European Resuscitation Council guidelines on http://www.erc.edu/).

Station 1.11 Anatomy: base of the skull

Information for the candidate

In this station you will be asked about the anatomy of the skull and structures passing through various foramen.

Examiner's mark sheet

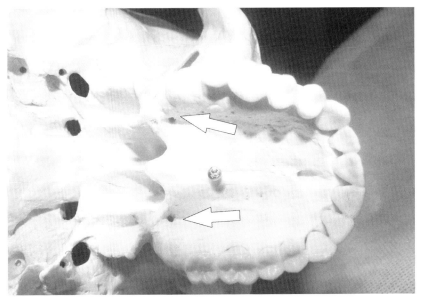

Figure 1.11a Palate.

marks

Name the foramen in Figure 1.11a
2 ☐

Greater palatine foramen.

What structures pass through this foramen?
1 ☐

Anterior (greater) palatine nerve and descending palatine vessels.

Name the foramen 5 in Figure 1.11b
1 ☐

Foramen ovale.

What structure passes through this?
1 ☐

Mandibular division of the trigeminal nerve (V3).

Name the foramen 4 in Figure 1.11b

2 ☐

Foramen rotundum.

What structure passes through this foramen?

1 ☐

Maxillary division of the trigeminal nerve (V2).

Which part of the face does this nerve provide sensory supply?

1 ☐

Over the cheek.

Does it supply any muscles?

1 ☐

No.

Indicate the carotid canal

2 ☐

The carotid canal is located in the temporal bone and it connects the base of the skull to the middle cranial fossa. The opening of the carotid canal in the middle cranial fossa is called the foramen lacerum (6 in Figure 1.11b). It contains the internal carotid artery and the sympathetic plexus surrounding the artery.

Indicate the optic canal

2 ☐

The optic foramen and canal are located at the base of the lesser wing of the sphenoid bone in the middle cranial fossa (2 in Figure 1.11b). It connects the middle cranial fossa to the orbit.

What does it contain?

2 ☐

It contains the optic nerve (II) and ophthalmic artery.

Name the foramen 9 in Figure 1.11b

2 ☐

Jugular foramen.

What structures pass through this?

2 ☐

Internal jugular vein, IX, X and XI nerves.

Total: /20

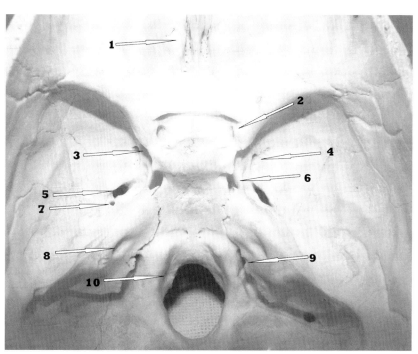

Figure 1.11b Base of the skull.

1. Cribriform plate; 2. Optic canal; 3. Superior orbital fissure; 4. Foramen rotundum; 5. Foramen ovale; 6. Foramen lacerum; 7. Foramen spinosum; 8. Internal acoustic meatus; 9. Jugular foramen; 10. Hypoglossal canal.

Table 1.11 Foramen in the base of the skull.

Foramen	Location	Content
Olfactory foramen	Cribriform plate of ethmoid	I nerve
Optic canal	Lesser wing of sphenoid	II nerve and ophthalmic artery
Superior orbital fissure	Between greater and lesser wing of sphenoid	III, IV, V1 and VI nerves
Foramen rotundum	Greater wing of sphenoid bone	V2 nerve
Foramen ovale	Sphenoid bone	V3 nerve and accessory meningeal artery
Foramen spinosum	Sphenoid bone	Nervus spinosus (branch of V3) and middle meningeal artery
Foramen lacerum	Temporal bone; opening of carotid canal in middle cranial fossa	Internal carotid artery and sympathetic plexus
Internal acoustic meatus	Temporal bone	VII, VIII nerves
Jugular foramen	Temporal and occipital bones	Internal jugular vein, IX, X and XI nerves
Hypoglossal canal	Occipital bone	XII nerve
Foramen magnum	Occipital bone	Spinal cord, meninges, vertebral arteries and veins
Stylomastoid foramen	Exterior: temporal bone	Facial nerve
Supra-orbital foramen	Face: frontal bone	Supra-orbital nerve, artery and vein

Table 1.11 Foramen in the base of the skull *continued:*

Foramen	Location	Content
Infra-orbital foramen	Face: maxillary bone	Infra-orbital nerve, artery and vein
Zygomatico-facial foramen	Face: zygomatic bone	Zygomatico-facial nerve
Mental foramen	Face: mandible	Mental nerve, artery and vein
Incisive foramen	Oral cavity: maxillary bone	Nasopalatine nerve, sphenopalatine artery and vein
Greater palatine foramen	Oral cavity: between maxillary and palatine bones	Greater palatine nerve, artery and vein
Lesser palatine foramen	Oral cavity: palatine bone	Lesser palatine nerve, artery and vein

V1= ophthalmic division of the trigeminal nerve
V2 = maxillary division of the trigeminal nerve
V3 = mandibular division of the trigeminal nerve

Key points

- The base of the skull is divided into three areas: the anterior, middle and posterior cranial fossae.
- There are several openings in the base of the skull which transmit cranial nerves and blood vessels.
- The three divisions of the trigeminal nerve (ophthalmic, maxillary and mandibular) exit the middle cranial fossa through the superior orbital fissure, foramen ovale and foramen rotundum.
- X, XI and XII cranial nerves exit the posterior cranial fossa via the jugular foramen.

Station 1.12 History taking: teeth extraction

Information for the candidate

In this station you will be asked to take a history from a 25-year-old male patient who is scheduled to have multiple teeth extraction.

Examiner's mark sheet

marks

Introduces him/herself to the patient.	1 ☐
Confirms the proposed surgery.	1 ☐
Past surgical history: elicits H/O previous anaesthetics.	1 ☐
Drug history: currently on methadone.	2 ☐
Dose of methadone 60mg daily.	1 ☐
H/O previous heroin abuse.	2 ☐
Route of heroin abuse (intravenous).	2 ☐
How long he has been using and when stopped (6 years; stopped 3 months ago).	2 ☐
H/O smoking: 20 cigarettes a day.	1 ☐
H/O alcohol intake: how much/what?	1 ☐
Past medical history: any hospital admission/medical problems (hepatitis 6 months ago).	2 ☐

H/O allergy: to egg.	1	[ ]
Type of allergic reaction (skin rash).	1	[ ]
H/O reflux and heartburn.	1	[ ]
Asks about dentures, crowns and caps (which tooth/teeth, is it loose?).	1	[ ]

Total:	/20

Information for the actor

You are scheduled to have your teeth extraction. You suffer from toothache and your dentist has suggested a tooth extraction. In the past you used to take intravenous heroin for 6 years; you stopped this about 3 months ago. To help with withdrawal symptoms you have been on methadone (30mg in the morning and another 30mg at night time) for the last 3 months. You are a little concerned about the pain during and after the operation. Apart from getting admitted for jaundice due to hepatitis 6 months ago, you do not have any other medical problems. You are allergic to eggs with which you get a rash. You still smoke cigarettes and drink alcohol. You have two (dental) crowns in the front on the upper jaw.

Information for the examiner

The patient has a past history of intravenous drug abuse (no longer abusing), a previous GA for appendicectomy as a child and no other history of note. A history of drug abuse is elicited when questioned about current medication. The patient may volunteer this information only when he is given an opportunity to express his concerns.

General principles for history taking

Time available for gathering all the necessary information is only 5 minutes. Therefore, it is important to have a structured approach. Read the given information carefully and plan your questions. If the information indicates that you take a history, you should not waste time in doing a clinical examination. You should gather information relevant to the clinical condition, as well as general questions that will help you to screen common medical conditions in the given patient. Allow the patient to outline their problem by using an open-ended question, but you should control the interview, so that 5 minutes of time is utilised appropriately.

Structured approach

- Introduce and confirm the patient's identity.
- Confirm the proposed surgical procedure, side and indication.
- Consider the presenting symptoms and whether they have any systemic effect.
- What is the cause of the current surgical condition, and does it have any systemic complications? Is there any predisposing or risk factor for the presenting problem?
- Past surgical history (PSH): previous anaesthetics, type of anaesthetic - any problems?
- Family history of anaesthetic-related concerns, diabetes and heart attack.
- Past medical history (PMH): previous hospital admissions, operations, visits to general practitioner, rheumatic fever, jaundice, high blood pressure, chest pain, heart attack, palpitations, cough, wheeze, dizziness, black-outs, stroke, jaundice, etc.
- Drugs: both for therapeutic and recreational purpose. Most women of reproductive age are likely to take the oral contraceptive pill and postmenopausal women may be taking hormone replacement therapy.
- Any side effects related to current drug therapy or any treatment the patient has received (e.g. radiotherapy, chemotherapy).
- Allergy: to drugs, food and other substances; type of reaction.
- History of smoking and alcohol.
- History of heartburn and gastrointestinal reflux.
- Mouth opening, crowns, caps, dentures, loose tooth.
- Neck stiffness, range of movement.

Systematic review (as directed by history)

Cardiovascular system: chest pain, shortness of breath, exercise tolerance, palpitation, dizziness or syncope (black out or faints) and ankle swelling.

Respiratory system: shortness of breath, wheeze, cough.

Central nervous system: headache, convulsions or fits, stroke (cerebrovascular accident), weakness, unsteady gait, paraesthesia, numbness, visual disturbances, mood changes (depression), memory loss and confusion.

Gastrointestinal system: heartburn, reflux, dysphagia, abdominal pain, jaundice, loss of appetite, change in bowel habit, melaena.

Locomotor system: arthritis (stiffness and joint pain), rheumatoid arthritis.

Endocrine system: thyroid disease, weight change, dislike to hot or cold weather, diarrhoea, constipation, palpitations, voice change, depression and tremors.

As you work through the questionnaire, if you identify a problem you can either ask a few questions pertaining to the problem and proceed with the remainder of the questionnaire, or you may first complete the questionnaire and then focus on areas of identified problems. Remember, 5 minutes is a short time and you need to be careful not to spend too much time on a specific issue and omit a big chunk, such as reflux and allergy, which may fetch you the marks.

Some patients may volunteer all information that is useful to you. Some may just be concerned about their current surgical problem and forget about all other significant medical problems that have been investigated and treated in the past. You may not elicit all the information unless you ask specific closed questions. If the patient has a history of jaundice or drug abuse, consider the possibility of hepatitis and AIDS.

Key points

- Whilst eliciting a drug history, do remember to ask about drugs for recreational purposes.
- When there is a positive past medical history (such as jaundice), try and find the cause for that (possibly it is due to intravenous drugs/ hepatitis in this case); it may lead to a series of relevant questions.
- Have a structure: introduction, confirmation of surgery, past surgical history, past medical history, family history, drugs, allergy, smoking and alcohol, dentures/mouth opening and neck range of movement.

Station 1.13 Simulation: anaphylaxis

Information for the candidate

A 70-year-old male patient is scheduled for a total hip replacement under general anaesthesia. He is a known hypertensive and is otherwise fit and healthy. He is now on the operating table.

On entering the station:

General anaesthesia was induced with propofol and fentanyl, and relaxation was facilitated with atracurium. The trachea was easily intubated; the lungs are ventilated with positive pressure ventilation. Just before starting the surgery the surgeon requested 1.5g of cefuroxime which was administered intravenously. Can you take over this patient for 5 minutes? You are the anaesthetist in charge for the next 5 minutes (surgery yet to be started). As you take over, the low saturation alarm and high airway pressure alarm sounds.

Examiner's mark sheet

marks

Checks other vital parameters and recognises this as a critical   1   ☐
incident.

Calls for help.   2   ☐

Administers 100% oxygen.   2 ☐

Checks the endotracheal tube position.   2 ☐

Auscultates the chest for breath sounds and any added sounds.   2 ☐

Mentions that he/she can hear a wheeze.   2 ☐

Asks for epinephrine/administers epinephrine 100μg IV.   2 ☐

Checks the intravenous drip and administers normal saline or   2 ☐
Hartmann's solution rapidly.

Looks for cutaneous signs of anaphylaxis such as rashes.   1 ☐

Asks for antihistamines: chlorpheniramine 10-20mg and   2 ☐
hydrocortisone 100mg to be administered intravenously.

Checks the response by reassessing the vital parameters and   2 ☐
repeats epinephrine if required.

Total:	/20

Information for the examiner

On SimMan, the heart rate is set at 130 per minute (sinus tachycardia), the high heart rate alarm is sounding, BP is set at 70/30 mmHg, peripheral pulses are very feeble and a carotid pulse is present. SaO_2 is low at 94%, $EtCO_2$ is low at 3.0kPa, end tidal isoflurane is 0.9, the high airway pressure alarm is sounding on the ventilator, the tidal volume is 500ml and the respiratory rate is 12 breaths per minute. The chest has bilateral wheezes and there is a reduced compliance of the chest on both sides.

As the candidates take over, the low saturation alarm and high airway pressure alarm sounds. Candidates should ask for a blood pressure reading to be taken (non-invasive blood pressure [NIBP] set at a 5-minute interval).

Recognition of anaphylaxis

In this scenario you should recognise an inadvertent high airway pressure, tachycardia and low oxygen saturation. Immediately check for other vital parameters: $EtCO_2$, blood pressure and a peripheral or central pulse. Diagnosis of anaphylaxis is based on the combination of the following clinical findings:

- Tachycardia.
- Hypotension.
- Severe bronchospasm.
- Low saturation indicating impaired gas exchange and reduced peripheral perfusion.
- Low $EtCO_2$ indicating reduced pulmonary perfusion.
- Unresponsiveness of haemodynamic parameters to initial treatment with ephedrine or metaraminol.

A systematic approach for recognition and management of this critical incident is very important.

Management of anaphylaxis

Primary therapy

- Stop administration of all agents likely to have caused the anaphylaxis.
- Call for help
- Maintain airway, give 100% oxygen and lie the patient flat with their legs elevated.
- Give epinephrine (adrenaline). This may be given intramuscularly in a dose of 0.5mg to 1mg (0.5-1ml of 1:1,000) and may be repeated every 10 minutes according to the arterial pressure and pulse, until improvement occurs. Alternatively, 50-100µg intravenously (0.5-1ml of 1:10,000) over 1 minute has been recommended for hypotension with titration of further doses as required.
- Start rapid intravenous infusion with colloids or crystalloids. Adult patients may require 2-4 litres of crystalloid.

Secondary therapy

- Give antihistamines (chlorpheniramine 10-20mg by slow intravenous infusion).
- Give corticosteroids (100-500mg hydrocortisone slow IV).
- Bronchodilators may be required for persistent bronchospasm.

Investigations

Serum tryptase: A blood sample should be collected as soon as possible after the initial management; about one hour after the reaction and about 6-24 hours after the reaction. The blood sample should be stored at 4°C if it can be analysed within 48 hours or should be stored at -20°C if there is a delay.

All events should be documented. All suspected anaphylactic reactions should be reported to the Committee on Safety of Medicine. After discharge from intensive care or the high dependency unit (HDU), the patient should be referred to an immunologist for further investigations.

(For further reading please refer to the Association of Anaesthetists of Great Britain and Ireland - Anaphylaxis guidelines).

Key points

- You should think about possible causes; the most likely cause is anaphylaxis.
- The scheduled surgical procedure is an elective one and the surgery has not commenced. So, it should be postponed.
- The most common substances causing anaphylactic reactions are neuromuscular blocking agents, latex, antibiotics, hypnotics, colloids and opioids (in decreasing order).
- The most common presentation under anaesthesia is cardiovascular (no pulse, tachycardia, hypotension) with bronchospasm.

Station 1.14 Monitoring equipment: capnography

Information for the candidate

In this station you will be asked about the methods of measuring expired CO_2 and interpretation of the display.

Examiner's mark sheet

marks

Can you identify this? 1 ☐

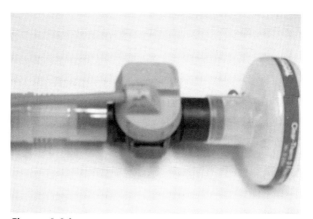

Figure 1.14a.

Main stream CO_2 analyser.

What other type of CO_2 analyser is used in clinical practice? 1 ☐

Side stream analyser.

What are the differences between the two?   4 ☐

Main stream

A cuvette containing a CO_2 sensor is inserted between the endotracheal tube (ETT) and breathing system. There is no need for gas sampling. Water vapour can condense on the sensor which can result in a false high reading. To overcome this, the sensor is heated to 39°C. It is heavier and cumbersome.

Side stream

The sensor is located in the main unit; gas is aspirated using a small pump via a sampling tube at a rate of 50-150ml/minute. As this gas also contains anaesthetic agent, it should be scavenged or returned to the patient's breathing system.

What are the advantages of a main stream analyser?   2 ☐

There is no delay in response, no loss in gas, and no mixing of sample gas with inspired gas.

Name the factors that can affect the response time   3 ☐

- The response time depends on transit time and rise time.
- Transit time depends on the length of the sample tube.
- Rise time depends on the optimum flow rate and the size of the sample chamber. A very low flow rate and large sample chamber increases the rise time.

Name the different phases of this capnograph in Figure 1.14b

4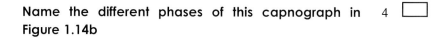

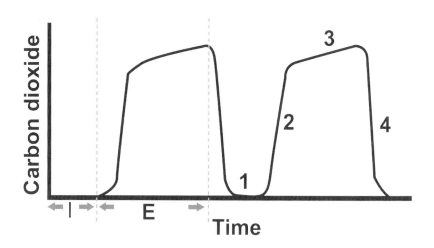

Figure 1.14b Normal capnograph.

1. Inspiratory base line: this should be at 0, since any elevation of the baseline indicates rebreathing.
2. Expiratory upslope phase: onset of expiration. If this is shallow it indicates obstruction.
3. Plateau: this represents mixing of alveolar gas; if sloped rather than flat, this indicates uneven mixing, as in chronic obstructive airway disease (COAD).
4. Fall to 0: inspiratory downstroke.

Name the following abnormal patterns of capnographs
5 ☐

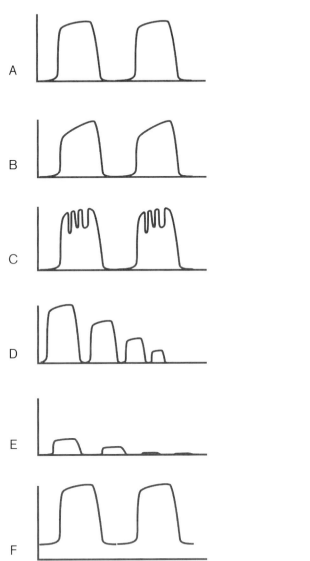

Figure 1.14c Patterns of capnographs.
A. Normal; B. Chronic obstructive airway disease; C. Curare cleft; D. Reduced cardiac output; E. Oesophageal intubation; F. Rebreathing.

Total: /20

Measurement of carbon dioxide

Capnometry is the measurement of CO_2 concentration during the respiratory cycle. Capnography is the graphic display of CO_2 concentration as a waveform, usually plotted as $EtCO_2$ versus time (CO_2 is plotted along the y axis and time along the x axis).

A capnograph uses the principle of infrared absorption by CO_2. Gases with molecules containing two or more different atoms absorb radiation in the infrared region of the spectrum. CO_2 has a strong absorption band at a wavelength of 4.26μm.

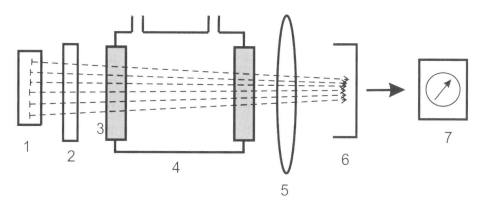

Figure 1.14d Infrared spectroscopy.
1. Infrared radiation source; 2. Filter; 3. Crystal window; 4. Sample chamber; 5. Focusing optics; 6. Photodetector; 7. Display.

The amount of infrared radiation absorbed is proportional to the CO_2 concentration. The electrical output from the photodetector is presented as partial pressure of CO_2 in the sample chamber.

A sudden decrease in the $EtCO_2$ value to near zero indicates a complete airway disconnection, totally obstructed airway or ventilator malfunction.

A sudden decrease in the $EtCO_2$ value to a low level (not near to zero) may be due to reduced cardiac output or a leak in the breathing system.

An exponential drop in $EtCO_2$ is usually as a result of reduced pulmonary perfusion due to low cardiac output or a pulmonary embolism.

A gradual decrease in $EtCO_2$ value indicates hyperventilation or hypothermia. Similarly, a gradual increase in $EtCO_2$ value indicates hypoventilation or increasing body temperature.

Key points

- There are two types of CO_2 analysers: side stream and main stream analysers.
- A main stream analyser adds additional weight to the breathing tubes and increases dead space.
- A side stream analyser is more convenient but there may be a delay in the response; the response time of the side stream analyser depends on transit time and rise time.

Station 1.15 Clinical safety: diathermy and electrical safety

Information for the candidate

In this station you will be tested on your knowledge and skills required to safely use clinical equipment.

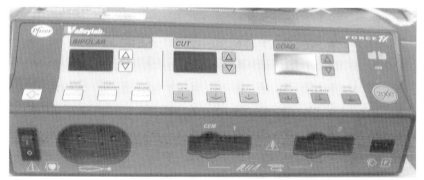

Figure 1.15a Diathermy machine.

Examiner's mark sheet

marks

What are the clinical uses of this equipment?   1 ☐

Diathermy involves employing high frequency alternating current to cut or to coagulate tissues during surgery.

What is the physical principle involved?   1 ☐

◆ High frequency current.
◆ Localised high density current.

What is the frequency of current used?   1 ☐

1MHz.

Why does the patient plate have a large area?   1 ☐

A large patient plate is to reduce the current density.

What happens if the patient plate is disconnected and diathermy is activated?   1 ☐

Current flows through the patient and is earthed through any metal objects which are attached to the patient.

Are there any other problems or hazards while using diathermy?   1 ☐

◆ Fire and explosion.
◆ Pacemaker dysfunction.

What is the difference between monopolar and bipolar diathermy?   2 ☐

Monopolar diathermy needs a patient (neutral) plate. Bipolar diathermy is like a pair of forceps where current travels down on one limb of the forceps and leaves through the other limb of the forceps. Bipolar diathermy delivers a lower power output.

What safety features are incorporated to avoid electrical hazards?

3

The outer case is earthed. An isolating capacitor provides high impedance to low frequency current. It has a floating circuit where the active electrode and neutral electrodes are isolated from the earth connection (earth-free circuit).

What precautions do you need to take to prevent electrical hazards (from diathermy) to the patient?

2 x 3
=6

A good connection of the neutral plate to the patient, not activating diathermy until the active electrode is in contact with the tissues and regular servicing of the equipment.

Figure 1.15b.

What does Figure 1.15b indicate?

2

Type CF equipment (leakage current is less than 10 micro-amperes).

Figure 1.15c.

What does Figure 1.15c indicate?   1 ☐

Type BF equipment. It provides a higher degree of protection against electric shock than that provided by Type B. Like Type CF, it is floating (identified by 'F') with respect to earth.

Total: /20

Key points

♦ Diathermy is an electrical device that utilises a heating effect of high frequency (0.5-1MHz) alternating current to cut and coagulate.

♦ A high frequency current is chosen to minimise the effects on cardiac and skeletal muscle.

♦ For cutting, a sine wave pattern is employed; for coagulation, a damped or pulse sine wave pattern is used.

♦ Current density is current per unit area. It is high at the diathermy forceps end and is low at the large earth plate (as in monopolar diathermy).

♦ Depending on the type of equipment, acceptable levels of leakage currents have been determined.

- B-type applied parts are non-cardiac grounded applied parts. These are parts that come into contact with the patient.
- C-type comes into contact with the heart. F stands for floating and is isolated. CF is for cardiac applications and provides a higher degree of protection against electric shock than BF.

Station 1.16 Radiology: chest X-ray

Information for the candidate

A 64-year-old male was admitted from the Accident and Emergency Department following polytrauma. Because of his open right supracondylar fracture he is posted for urgent open reduction and internal fixation. In view of his chest pain a chest X-ray was taken.

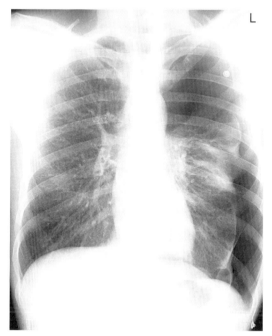

Figure 1.16a Chest X-ray.

Examiner's mark sheet

Please tick the correct answer - true or false.   **marks**

1. X-ray shows a right-sided pneumothorax.   True False 2 ☐
2. The findings are suggestive of tension True False 2 ☐
   pneumothorax.
3. There are fractured ribs with flail segments.   True False 2 ☐
4. If clinically deteriorating, immediate management is True False 2 ☐
   intubation and intermittent positive pressure
   ventilation (IPPV) with 100% oxygen.
5. His cardiothoracic ratio is within acceptable limits. True False 2 ☐
6. There is evidence for a right-sided haemothorax.   True False 2 ☐
7. A supraclavicular brachial plexus block is safe for True False 2 ☐
   his proposed surgery.
8. General anaesthesia with oxygen/nitrous True False 2 ☐
   oxide/sevoflurane and spontaneous ventilation will
   be a good choice.
9. This patient may have chronic obstructive airway True False 2 ☐
   disease.
10. In a normal chest X-ray you may see 6 ribs True False 2 ☐
    anteriorly and 10 ribs posteriorly.

Total: /20

Answers

1. False. Left-sided pneumothorax.

2. False. There is no tracheal or mediastinal shift.

3. False. There is no obvious bony injury.

4. False. Immediate management is decompression with a wide-bore
   needle in the second intercostal space in the midclavicular line.

5. True. It is <0.5.

6. False. The costophrenic and cardiophrenic angles are free in the right side.

7. False. There is a risk of pneumothorax and may result in bilateral pneumothoraces.

8. False. Nitrous oxide can increase the size of air-containing cavities.

9. True. There are features of hyperinflation of lung fields.

10. True.

Cardiothoracic ratio

Cardiothoracic ratio: this is a measurement to determine the size of the heart and a screening for heart enlargement.

ID: greatest internal diameter of the thorax.

MRD: maximum transverse diameter of the right side of the heart; it is a line drawn from the midline of the spine to the most distant point of the right cardiac margin.

MLD: maximum transverse diameter of the left side of the heart; it is a line drawn from the midline of the spine to the most distant point of the left cardiac margin.

Cardiothoracic ratio = MRD + MLD / ID.

Borders of the heart in a chest X-ray

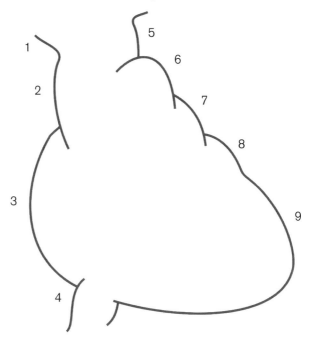

Figure 1.16b Borders of the heart.
1. Brachiocephalic vein; 2. Superior vena cava; 3. Right atrium; 4. Inferior vena cava; 5. Left subclavian artery; 6. Aortic knob; 7. Main pulmonary artery; 8. Left atrial appendage; 9. Left ventricle.

Key points

- The normal cardiothoracic ratio is less than 0.5.
- Tension pneumothorax is a clinical diagnosis.
- The presence of mediastinal shift and tracheal deviation to the opposite side may indicate a tension pneumothorax.

Station 1.17 History taking: arthroscopy of the knee

Information for the candidate

In the following station you will be asked to take a history from a patient who is scheduled to have arthroscopy of the knee as a day-case procedure.

Examiner's mark sheet

	marks	
Introduces him/herself to the patient.	1	☐
Confirms the proposed surgery.	1	☐
H/O trauma 3 days ago (fall while playing football).	2	☐
H/O previous anaesthetic.	1	☐
H/O heart murmur.	2	☐
Diagnosed at the age of 5.	1	☐
Had an echo at the age of 10, which showed a small ventricular septal defect (VSD); surgical correction was not required.	2	☐
Good exercise tolerance.	2	☐
H/O mild asthma, not precipitated by NSAIDs.	2	☐
Drug history: cocodamol for pain; salbutamol metered dose inhaler as and when required.	2	☐
H/O allergy: none known.	1	☐
H/O smoking: 15-20 cigarettes per day.	1	☐

H/O alcohol intake: 6-8 units on weekends.   1   ☐

Asks about dentures, crowns and caps.   1   ☐

Total:	/20

Information for the actor

You are 25 years old. Three days ago you injured your knee while playing football. Now you require keyhole surgery on the left knee joint. You know that you have a heart murmur. This was diagnosed when you were about 5 years old. You had a heart scan and were told that a small hole in the heart is causing the murmur. You did not require any further treatment. You also have mild asthma for which you take salbutamol via an inhaler when required. You also occasionally take tablets such as ibuprofen for headache.

For the last 3 days you have been taking painkillers (cocodamol). You smoke about 15-20 cigarettes per day, and drink alcohol only at the weekends.

Key points

◆ Ensure that all key symptoms have been elicited.
◆ Enquire as to the reason for arthroscopy and the nature of injury.
◆ Remember to ask complete details regarding the asthma and heart murmur.
◆ Ensure that it is safe to use NSAIDs during the peri-operative period in this patient.

(For more information please refer to OSCE set 1, station 1.12).

Station 1.18 Communication: awareness under anaesthesia

Information for the candidate

The nurse from the orthopaedic ward bleeps you to come and see a patient you anaesthetised one week ago. You put him to sleep for multiple long-bone fracture fixations following polytrauma in an emergency list when you were on-call. He claims that he was awake during his operation. He is upset.

Examiner's mark sheet

	marks	
Introduces him/herself to the patient.	1	☐
Discusses in the presence of a witness, e.g. a ward nurse.	1	☐
Confirms the facts, listens to the history, finds out what he actually does recollect.	2	☐
Offers an apology.	1	☐
Advises the patient that all precautionary measures, including a machine check, choice of drugs, monitoring, etc. were taken.	2	☐
As he was unstable following polytrauma, until he was stabilised you had to be careful with administration of drugs. It was possibly during that period that he had awareness.	2	☐
Finds out whether he felt pain during his awareness.	1	☐
Mentions that this is rare, but a possible complication whilst anaesthetising unstable trauma patients.	1	☐
Arranges an interview with a senior consultant.	2	☐

Offers follow-up.   1 ☐

Offers to organise psychological support.   2 ☐

Reassures that in the future general anaesthetics can be   1 ☐
safely provided.

Advises him that everything is documented and you will write   1 ☐
to his GP.

Enquires as to whether he wants to know anything more.   1 ☐

Remains courteous and develops rapport.   1 ☐

Total: /20

Information for the actor

You are Mr. AM. A week ago you were brought to the hospital following a motor vehicle accident. You were quite poorly and had lost a lot of blood. You underwent an operation to fix all your bone fractures. You remember the anaesthetist putting the tube into the windpipe and taking you to the theatre. During this you felt as though you were not able to breathe. You were upset because something went wrong with the anaesthetic and you woke up half way through the operation just like you watched on the television a while ago. You wish to speak to the anaesthetist involved to find out what exactly went wrong. You are upset and worried that the same thing may happen again in case you ever need any further operations.

Awareness under anaesthesia

Awareness during anaesthesia can be deliberate (as in regional techniques or during spinal surgeries where patients are woken up in the middle of the procedure - intentionally). Inadvertent awareness during anaesthesia can either be an explicit or implicit memory.

Awareness with an explicit memory can be conscious awareness with recall, with or without pain. In an implicit memory type, there is an apparent perception during anaesthesia without conscious awareness or recall.

Enquire as to the possibility of getting confused with dreaming or delirium (as with ketamine).

The risk of awareness is possibly higher in:

◆ Obstetrics and trauma (shocked) patients.
◆ Total intravenous anaesthesia (due to technical failures or inadequate drugs).

It can also be due to human error, erroneous clinical judgement or, technical faults.

Key points

When there is a complaint on awareness under anaesthesia:

◆ Patients can be furious; remain courteous, professional and objective.
◆ See the patient as early as you can.
◆ Have a ward nurse or some other responsible personnel present when you discuss this with the patient.
◆ Apologising does not imply accepting guilt. But it goes a long way.
◆ Get the facts right, listen to the patient; do not be defensive.
◆ Find out what exactly they recall, when they were aware and whether they were experiencing pain at that time; rule out dreaming or delirium.
◆ Give them a good explanation on the conduct of anaesthesia, and the precautions and safety measures taken to avoid awareness, e.g. machine check, alarms, monitor, clinical evaluation, etc.
◆ Most hospitals have a consultant with a special interest in awareness under anaesthesia.
◆ Reassure about future anaesthetics.
◆ Offer psychological support if they develop post-traumatic stress disorder.
◆ Document and communicate with the appropriate doctors, including the GP.

Station 1.19 Anatomy: intercostal nerve block

Information for the candidate

In this station you will be assessed on anatomy of the intercostal space and the technique of intercostal nerve block.

Examiner's mark sheet

marks

Name the structures labelled 1 to 7 in Figure 1.19a   1 x 7 ☐

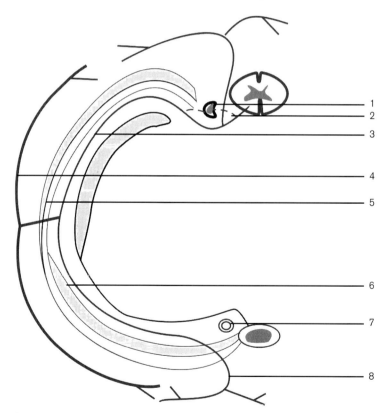

Figure 1.19a Intercostal nerve.
1. Sympathetic ganglia; 2. Rami communicantes; 3. Intercostal nerve; 4. Lateral cutaneous branch; 5. External intercostal muscle; 6. Internal intercostal muscle; 7. Internal mammary artery; 8. Anterior cutaneous branch.

Which are the three important structures passing through the intercostal space? How are they arranged? 3 ☐

Intercostal vein, artery and nerve (VAN), from above downwards.

How many veins are there in each space? 2 ☐

One posterior and two anterior veins.

Give three indications for intercostal nerve block 3 ☐

Thoracic surgery, breast surgery, upper abdominal procedures such as cholecystectomy, rib fractures, intercostal drain insertion.

Between which two muscles are these intercostal nerves and vessels found? 1 ☐

The neurovascular bundle is found between the internal intercostal and innermost intercostal muscles.

State three complications of intercostal nerve block 3 ☐

Pneumothorax, intravascular injection, bleeding, nerve damage and local anaesthetic toxicity.

What type of nerve is the intercostal nerve? 1 ☐

Mixed spinal nerve.

Total: /20

Intercostal nerves

The T1 to T12 spinal nerves, after emerging from the intervertebral foramina divide into an anterior and posterior division. The posterior division provides sensory and motor innervation to the paravertebral region.

Each nerve is connected to the sympathetic chain that lies antero-lateral to the vertebral body through the white and gray rami communicantes.

The anterior division continues along the intercostal space as the intercostal nerve. It runs in the costal groove on the inner surface of the inferior border of the body of the rib. The costal groove provides a protective function to the neurovascular bundle.

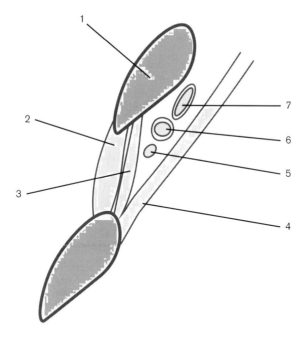

Figure 1.19b Intercostal space.
1. Rib; 2. External intercostal muscle; 3. Internal intercostal muscle; 4. Innermost intercostal muscle; 5. Intercostal nerve; 6. Intercostal artery; 7. Intercostal vein.

The intercostal nerve gives rise to a lateral cutaneous branch (anterior to the mid-axillary line) and an anterior cutaneous branch closer to the midline.

T1 sends fibres to the upper limb. T2 contributes to the intercostobrachial nerve. T3 to T6 supply the thorax and the remainder innervate the abdominal wall. T11 and I12 are described as subcostal nerves.

Intercostal nerve blocks are performed for chest wall procedures and upper abdominal procedures. They do not provide visceral analgesia. Therefore, for upper abdominal surgeries it needs to be combined with a coeliac plexus block for complete analgesia.

In view of the vascularity, intercostal nerve blocks have a high propensity to cause local anaesthetic toxicity, in particular, when multiple level injections are done. The peak plasma level occurs more rapidly and is higher following intercostal nerve block than from other regional nerve blocks when comparable doses are injected.

The optimal site for blocking an intercostal nerve is at the angle of the rib and the optimal needle is one with a short bevel.

Key points

♦ Intercostal nerve blocks are performed to provide analgesia for thoracic and upper abdominal procedures.
♦ Due to high vascularity, there is an increased risk of local anaesthetic toxicity.

Station 1.20 Clinical examination: cranial nerves

Information for the candidate

In this station you will be asked to perform cranial nerve examination on a volunteer.

Examiner's mark sheet

marks

Olfactory nerve Asks about smell. 1 ☐

Optic nerve Visual acuity: light reflex in both eyes and indirect light reflex. 2 ☐

Oculomotor, trochlear and abducens nerves Checks eye movements in all four directions. 2 ☐

What nerves do you test by light reflex? 2 ☐

II (optic) and III (oculomotor).

Trigeminal nerve Checks sensation over the face and forehead. 1 ☐

Clenching teeth for masseter and temporalis muscles. 1 ☐

Facial nerve
Special senses: asks about taste 1 ☐
Motor: asks the patient to shut their eyes tightly; smile/show teeth/blow out their cheeks. 1 ☐

Vestibulocochlear nerve Hearing. 2 ☐

Glossopharyngeal nerve Gag reflex (not necessary to test). 1 ☐

Vagus nerve Movement of soft palate (on saying 'Ha'). 1 ☐

Accessory nerve Shrugging the shoulders. 1 ☐

Hypoglossal nerve Look for tongue wasting/fasciculations. 1 ☐

State the signs of complete paralysis of the third cranial nerve

3 ☐

Ptosis, the eye is displaced downwards and outwards, the pupil is dilated and there is a loss of accommodation reflex.

Total: /20

Summary of cranial nerve function

- I - Smell.
- II - Visual acuity, visual fields and ocular fundi.
- II, III - Pupillary reactions.
- III, IV, VI - Extra-ocular movements, including opening of the eyes.
- V - Facial sensation, movements of the jaw, and corneal reflexes.
- VII - Facial movements and gustation.
- VIII - Hearing and balance.
- IX, X - Swallowing, elevation of the palate and gag reflex.
- V, VII, X, XII - Voice and speech.
- XI - Shrugging the shoulders and turning the head.
- XII - Movement and protrusion of the tongue.

In this station it is unrealistic to expect you to formally examine all 12 cranial nerves. Examination of olfaction, gag reflex, etc., will be restricted to simple questions.

Olfactory nerve

Ensure patency of the nostrils. Each nostril should be tested separately, occluding the other one, with the eyes closed.

Optic nerve

First, visual acuity is examined by asking the patient to read a pocket visual acuity chart. Each eye is tested separately with the other eye covered. Then, visual fields are tested by a confrontation test. The examiner sits facing the patient at eye level. When the right eye is being examined ask the patient to cover his/her left eye with the left hand and vice versa.

Assess the diameter and equality of pupils. Shine a light and assess the direct and consensual light reflex. A pupillary reflex tests optic and oculomotor nerves. An accommodation reflex can be tested by bringing an object closer to the eye and assessing pupillary size. Eyes accommodate to nearer objects by constricting the pupils.

Oculomotor, trochlear and abducens nerves

These nerves supply the extra-ocular muscles. The trochlear nerve supplies superior oblique (SO4); the abducens nerve supplies lateral rectus (LR6); the remainder are supplied by the oculomotor nerve. These nerves are tested by asking the patient to follow the moving fingers of the examiner without moving his/her head.

The oculomotor nerve also supplies levator palpebrae, the elevator of the eyelids. Third nerve palsy can cause ptosis. Parasympathetic fibres run along with the third nerve, hence third nerve palsy is associated with disruption of parasympathetic activity as well, resulting in pupillary dilatation (sympathetics dilate the pupil and parasympathetics constrict the pupil).

Trigeminal nerve

The trigeminal nerve supplies the muscles of mastication and sensory innervation for the face. Motor supply is tested by feeling for the masseter and temporalis muscle tone after asking the patient to clench their teeth (pterygoids).

Sensory innervation is tested in all three distributions: ophthalmic, maxillary and mandibular divisions. Commonly, pin prick (with a blunt point), fine touch (with cotton wool), and warm and cold modalities are tested.

The corneal reflex involves testing V and VII nerves. With a wisp of cotton touch the cornea. Observe for reflex blinking.

Facial nerve

Look for creases in the forehead, the nasolabial groove, facial asymmetry, etc. The common tests for this nerve include raising the eyebrows (frown), shutting the eyes tight, saying 'E' or smiling to show the teeth, and by trying to blow air with the lips tightly closed (puff out cheeks).

If the lesion in the nerve is peripheral it results in weakness involving the entire half of the face on the involved side. If it is a central lesion, the upper half of the face is spared (as this part receives dual innervation from both hemispheres).

Vestibulocochlear nerve

Although the nerve is important for hearing and balance, at the bed-side, hearing is often tested to identify any lesion. Because of extensive bilateral connection of the auditory system and practical limitations, precise diagnosis of the nature and side of the lesion of the nerve is difficult.

With the patient's eyes closed, in a calm environment, hearing is tested on both sides with sounds, such as ticking of the watch, rubbing of the fingers, etc. Patients should identify whether they hear it in the right or left side. If a tuning fork is provided, Weber (for lateralisation) and Rinne (for air versus bone conduction) tests can be done. Normally, air conduction is greater than bone conduction. If there is a suspicion about hearing impairment, an audiogram should be requested for further evaluation.

Glossopharyngeal and vagus nerves

Both the nerves are tested together. Enquire as to whether the patient has any hoarseness of voice or difficulty in swallowing. Ask the patient to say 'Aah' and look for movement of the pharynx and soft palate. Normally, the uvula remains in the midline and the soft palate rises symmetrically on both sides. In a unilateral lesion, the uvula is drawn to the normal side.

The gag reflex (sensory IX motor X) is tested by stimulating the pharynx (back of throat) on both sides. A normal response is a gag or cough.

Accessory nerve

The accessory nerve innervates trapezius and the sternocleidomastoid muscles. Apart from observing for wasting of these muscles (trapezius from behind), the nerves can be tested by asking the patient to shrug the shoulders against resistance (for trapezius) and by turning the head towards the opposite side against resistance (for sternocleidomastoid).

Hypoglossal nerve

The hypoglossal nerve supplies the intrinsic muscles of the tongue and is tested by asking the patient to protrude his tongue. Normally, it is a sharp protrusion with the tongue remaining in the midline. Look for fasciculations, wasting or deviation. A unilateral lesion causes deviation of the tongue towards the affected side.

Key points

◆ A visual field test and reaction of the pupil to light tests the optic nerve.
◆ Normal eye movement in all directions indicates normal function of the 3rd, 4th and 6th cranial nerves.
◆ The muscles of facial expression are supplied by the 7th cranial nerve.
◆ 9th and 10th nerve function are tested by the gag reflex.
◆ Paralysis of the 12th cranial nerve causes deviation of the tongue towards the paralysed side.

OSCE
set 2

Station 2.1 Anaesthetic equipment: Humphrey ADE breathing system

Information for the candidate

In this station you will be asked questions with regards to a breathing system.

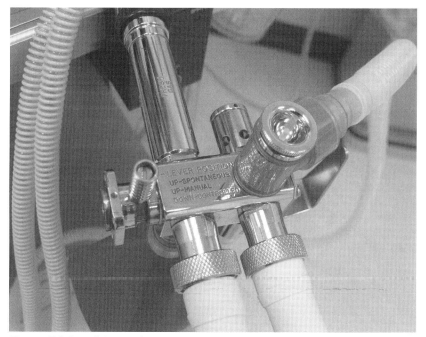

Figure 2.1 Breathing system.

Examiner's mark sheet

marks

What is this equipment?

2 ☐

Humphrey's ADE breathing system.

Name the various components of this system

4 ☐

- Inspiratory and expiratory tubing.
- Humphrey block which consists of an APL valve with indicator and a reservoir bag.
- Lever to select a spontaneous or controlled mode.
- Ventilator connection port and safety pressure relief valve.

At what pressure does the safety valve open?

2 ☐

$60cmH_2O$.

What are the advantages of this system?

4 ☐

- It is an efficient system both for spontaneous and controlled ventilation.
- A single system for adult and children.
- Choice of technique: as a semi-closed system without the soda lime canister or, as a circle system with the canister.
- Easy scavenging.

Explain the mechanism of its action

4 ☐

It acts as a Mapleson A system (Magill) when the lever is turned up. When the lever is turned down it acts as a Mapleson E system for controlled ventilation.

What is the fresh gas flow (FGF) required during spontaneous ventilation?   2   ☐

50-60ml/Kg/min.

What is the FGF required during controlled ventilation?   2   ☐

70ml/Kg/min.

| Total: | /20 |

Humphrey ADE system

The Humphrey ADE system can be converted into a Mapleson A to D or E by selecting the lever position. For spontaneous ventilation it is used as a Mapleson A and for controlled ventilation it is used as a Mapleson E system.

With the lever turned up, it works in Mapleson A mode. The reservoir bag on the ADE block is connected to the inspiratory limb. Expired gas passes through the expiratory limb to an APL valve to which scavenging can be connected. During the end of expiration, a mixture of alveolar and dead space gas escapes through the APL valve. During the inspiratory phase, gas is breathed in from the inspiratory limb and reservoir bag.

With the lever turned down, the reservoir bag is isolated from the inspiratory limb and the APL valve is isolated from the expiratory limb. The whole system acts as a T-piece system, the inspiratory limb acts as a gas delivery tube to the patient end of the T-piece and the expiratory limb acts as a reservoir limb of the T-piece. This is now a Mapleson E system. By attaching a reservoir bag and APL valve to this limb it can be converted to a Mapleson D system. The expiratory limb (reservoir tube of the T-piece) can be connected to a bag squeezer-type ventilator and it can be used for controlled ventilation.

Key points

- ◆ The Humphrey ADE system functions as a Mapleson A system with the lever in the up position.
- ◆ It functions as a Mapleson E system with the lever in the down position.
- ◆ It is suitable for both adult and paediatric use.
- ◆ It is an efficient system, both for spontaneous and controlled ventilation.

Station 2.2 Data interpretation: ECG

Information for the candidate

A 70-year-old male patient is scheduled for repair of a left inguinal hernia. There is a history of angina and syncope on exertion.

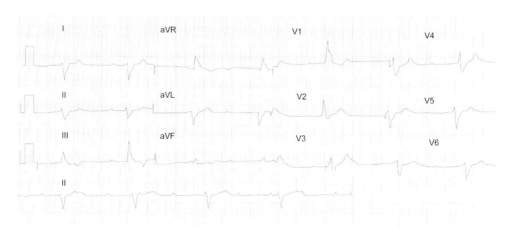

Figure 2.2 ECG.

Examiner's mark sheet

Please tick the correct answer - true or false.   **marks**

1. Standardisation in this ECG is 5mm = 1mV.   True   False   2 ☐
2. Normal recording speed is 50mm per second.   True   False   2 ☐
3. The heart rate in this ECG is approximately 75   True   False   2 ☐
    beats per minute.
4. This ECG shows a first degree heart block.   True   False   2 ☐
5. There is right bundle branch block (RBBB).   True   False   2 ☐
6. Limit of the normal cardiac axis is -30° to +90° True   False   2 ☐
7. There is right axis deviation.   True   False   2 ☐
8. This could be due to fibrosis of the bundle of His. True False 2 ☐
9. This could be due to block in the left anterior True   False   2 ☐
    descending (left inter-ventricular artery) branch of
    the LCA.
10. This patient may need cardiac pacing prior to   True   False   2 ☐
    surgery.

Total: /20

Answers

1. False. 10mm = 1mV.

2. False. 25mm/second.

3. False. Ventricular rate is about 40/minute.

4. False. Complete heart block.

5. True.

   ◆ Typical RBBB: QRS duration >120ms; rSR' or rsR' pattern in lead V1;
      wide terminal S wave in leads I and V6.
   ◆ Typical LBBB: QRS duration >120ms; upright (monophasic) QRS in
      leads I and V6; predominantly negative QRS complex in lead V1.

6. True.

7. True. Normally, the depolarisation waves spread in the heart so that the QRS deflections are positive in II and negative in aVR. In general, the axis can be identified by looking at QRS deflections in leads I, II and III. In a normal axis, all three will show positive deflection. In right axis deviation, the deflection in I becomes negative (downward) and the deflection in III becomes positive (upwards). In left axis deviation, the QRS is predominantly negative in III. (But, left axis deviation is not 'significant' until QRS deflection is negative in II as well).

8. True.

9. True.

10. True.

ECG criteria in complete heart block

◆   QRS: generally normal looking. When block occurs at the AV node or bundle of His, the QRS complex will appear normal. When block occurs at bundle branch level, the QRS complex will be widened.
◆   P waves: normal.
◆   Rate: the atrial rate will be unaffected by third degree AV block. The ventricular rate will be slower than the atrial rate. With intranodal third degree AV block, the ventricular rate is usually 40 to 60 beats/minute; with infranodal third degree AV block, the ventricular rate is usually less than 40 beats/minute.
◆   Rhythm: the atrial rhythm is usually regular, although sinus arrhythmia may be present. The ventricular rhythm will be regular.
◆   PR interval: since the atria and ventricles are depolarised from different pacemakers, they are independent of each other, and the PR interval will vary.

This patient needs to be referred to a cardiologist for the insertion of a pacemaker prior to having his surgery.

The following are indications for a pacemaker:

- Sinus node: sick sinus syndrome, recurrent Stoke-Adams syndrome, sinus node dysfunction.
- Conduction system: complete heart block, symptomatic second dogroo hoart block, symptomatic bifascicular and trifascicular heart block.
- Chronic atrial fibrillation.
- Persistent and symptomatic second- or third degree AV block associated with myocardial infarction.
- Atrio-biventricular pacing in moderate to severe heart failure.

Key points

- In complete heart block, the P wave and QRS complex are independent of each other.
- A normal axis is between +90 to -30°.
- Left anterior hemi-block is suspected in the presence of left axis deviation.
- The left bundle branch usually receives blood from the left anterior descending artery.

Station 2.3 Data interpretation: drug overdose

Information for the candidate

A 35-year-old female patient presented to an emergency department with a history of a drug overdose. Circumstances suggest that she has probably consumed drugs about two hours ago. She has been previously admitted with a drug overdose and has a history of depression for which she is on regular fluoxetine 40mg once daily. She complains of headache, terrible buzzing in her head, and mild deafness. The following are the results of blood toots porformod on arrival.

◆ PaO_2: 13kPa, $PaCO_2$: 3.7kPa, pH: 7.48, HCO_3^-: 18mmol/L.

◆ Na^+: 141mmol/L, K^+: 3.0mmol/L, Cl^-: 98mmol/L, glucose: 5.0mmol/L.

◆ Plasma salicylate level: 8.5mmol/L.

◆ Urea: 5.6mmol/L, creatinine: 70µmol/L.

Based on the above blood results answer the following questions.

Examiner's mark sheet

Please tick the correct answer - true or false.   **marks**

1. Activated charcoal will be useful.   True   False   2 ☐
2. Forced alkaline diuresis aids increased elimination   True   False   2 ☐
   of salicylates.
3. The above pH can be explained by associated   True   False   2 ☐
   metabolic alkalosis.
4. This patient has compensatory respiratory alkalosis.   True   False   2 ☐
5. This patient may need haemodialysis.   True   False   2 ☐
6. A recognised cause of death in salicylate poisoning   True   False   2 ☐
   is non-cardiogenic pulmonary oedema.
7. Acidosis is a poor prognostic sign in salicylate   True   False   2 ☐
   poisoning.
8. The anion gap is reduced in salicylate poisoning.   True   False   2 ☐
9. Chronic salicylate intoxication is easier to diagnose   True   False   2 ☐
   than acute intoxication.
10. The anion gap in this patient is 20mmol/L.   True   False   2 ☐

Total:	/20

Answers

1. True. Activated charcoal is indicated if an adult presents with a salicylate overdose of more than 250mg/Kg within one hour of ingestion. Gastric absorption after ingestion of a high dosage of salicylates is slow and hence gastric lavage and activated charcoal may be effective up to 24 hours.

2. True. Acidic drugs are eliminated best in alkaline urine. Urinary alkalinisation is achieved with 1.26% sodium bicarbonate. Increased elimination is indicated when plasma levels exceed 3.6mmol/L. Forced diuresis is not a commonly recommended treatment now because of other complications, such as pulmonary oedema.

3. False. It is because of respiratory alkalosis. A mixed respiratory alkalosis with metabolic acidosis with a normal or increased pH is a common presentation in adults.

4. False. Respiratory alkalosis is the primary acid-base disorder. It results from direct respiratory centre stimulation.

5. True. Haemodialysis is the treatment for severe poisoning and is considered in patients with a plasma salicylate concentration of more than 5.1mmol/L or a lower concentration associated with significant metabolic or clinical features. Normally, aspirin is 90% protein bound; in overdose, more than 25% in plasma is free and can be removed by haemodialysis.

6. True. Non-cardiogenic pulmonary oedema, disseminated intravascular coagulation (DIC), deranged clotting, low platelets, haematemesis, hyperpyrexia, hypoglycaemia, hypokalaemia and renal failure are potentially lethal uncommon presentations.

7. True.

8. False. Wide anion-gap.

9. False. Symptoms are non-specific.

10. False. Anion gap = $(Na^+ + K^+) - (Cl^- + HCO_3^-) = (141+3) - (98+18) = $ 28mmol/L.

Key points

◆   Aspirin is a weak acid and is more ionised in alkaline pH.
◆   Salicylate at a dose <150mg/Kg is unlikely to cause toxicity, 150-300mg/Kg produces moderate toxicity, >500mg/Kg can cause severe toxicity.
◆   Common presentation includes vomiting and dehydration, vertigo, tinnitus and deafness, warm extremities with sweating, tachypnoea and hyperventilation, along with acid-base disturbances.
◆   Although the plasma level does not necessarily correspond to toxicity, in general, toxicity is associated with a plasma level >2.5mmol/L.

Station 2.4 Data interpretation: neuro-observation chart

Information for the candidate

The chart (Figure 2.4) belongs to a 47-year-old male patient involved in a road traffic accident who has sustained a severe head injury. The CT scan is suggestive of diffuse axonal injury and revealed a large contusion in the occipital region. He has been ventilated in the ICU for the last 24 hours.

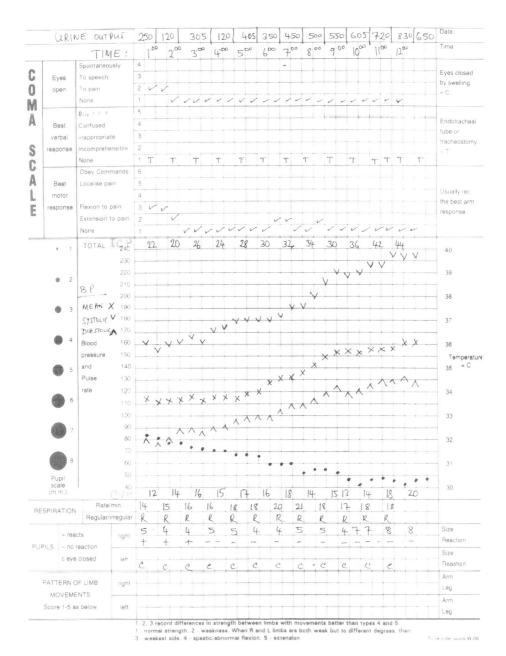

Figure 2.4 Neuro-observation chart.

x: mean blood pressure; v: systolic blood pressure; ^: diastolic blood pressure;
●: heart rate; CVP: central venous pressure; ICP: intracranial pressure.

Examiner's mark sheet

Please tick the correct answer - true or false.   **marks**

1. The Glasgow coma scale is very useful in this   True False 2 ☐
    patient now.
2. Intravenous 10% mannitol should be administered True False 2 ☐
    slowly to this patient.
3. A beta blocker would be useful to control the   True False 2 ☐
    hypertension.
4. The cause of hypertension is likely to be due to a True False 2 ☐
    decreased level of sedation.
5. At 7.00 hours his cerebral perfusion pressure was True False 2 ☐
    80 mmHg.
6. Urinary osmolality will be greater than True False 2 ☐
    350mOsmol/Kg.
7. Urinary sodium will be high in this patient.   True False 2 ☐
8. This patient's plasma sodium is likely to be less True False 2 ☐
    than 140mmol/L.
9. Use of 1-desamino-8-D arginine vasopressin True False 2 ☐
    (DDAVP) is indicated in this patient.
10. Use of dextrose-containing intravenous fluids are True False 2 ☐
    absolutely contra-indicated in this patient.

Total:	/20

Answers

1. False. Although the GCS is useful in the immediate assessment and
    to assess prognosis, it is unlikely to be of much help at this stage in a
    ventilated patient.

2. False. Mannitol is only useful in certain circumstances where definitive
    management to address an increase in ICP (such as neurosurgical

intervention) is planned. It will be of no benefit for this patient. When administered, mannitol is given rapidly.

3. False. Already the heart rate is low; beta-blockers may not be an ideal drug of choice.

4. False. Hypertension with bradycardia is unlikely to be due to emergence from sedation.

5. False. Cerebral perfusion pressure = MAP - ICP; at 7:00 hours it should have been: 130 - 32 = 98 mmHg.

6. False. Diabetes insipidus is a recognised complication of brain injury in which the concentrating ability of the kidney is lost due to a deficiency of vasopressin (anti-diuretic hormone), resulting in poorly concentrated urine.

7. False. Low.

8. False. Because of renal water loss, plasma sodium becomes concentrated and the level increases.

9. True. DDAVP (desmopressin) is a synthetic vasopressin analogue.

10. False. Dextrose-containing solutions, if possible, are best avoided. Once dextrose is metabolised in the body, it leaves behind either plain water or a hypotonic saline solution. Water passes into the brain cells thereby causing intracellular oedema and poor neurological recovery. However, if the patient is hypoglycaemic, a glucose-containing solution can be used.

The clinical features in the given scenario are suggestive of a terminal stage of head injury. This patient has hypertension and bradycardia, a phenomenon described by Harvey Cushing in 1902, known as Cushing's reflex. Ischaemia of the hypothalamus activates the sympathetic system, increases myocardial contractility, heart rate and vasoconstriction. This increases blood pressure and maintains cerebral perfusion. Raised blood pressure increases baroreceptor discharge, inhibiting the vasomotor centre, which in turn increases parasympathetic discharge, resulting in bradycardia.

This patient has a high urine output suggestive of diabetes insipidus. Other features of diabetes insipidus include low urine osmolality (50-200mOsm/Kg), high serum osmolality and normal-to-elevated serum sodium. Urine output usually is greater than 90ml/Kg/day (~4ml/Kg/hour), with a specific gravity of less than 1.010. Trauma and surgery around the region of the pituitary and hypothalamus are common causes of diabetes insipidus. It is treated with subcutaneous, nasal, and oral preparations of vasopressin analogues (DDAVP).

Key points

◆ Cushing's reflex is hypertension and bradycardia in the presence of increased intracranial tension.
◆ Diabetes insipidus is a recognised complication of severe head injury.
◆ Diabetes insipidus is characterised by high urine output, low urine osmolality and high or normal serum osmolality.

Station 2.5 Anatomy: stellate ganglion

Information for the candidate

In this station you will be asked questions on stellate ganglion block.

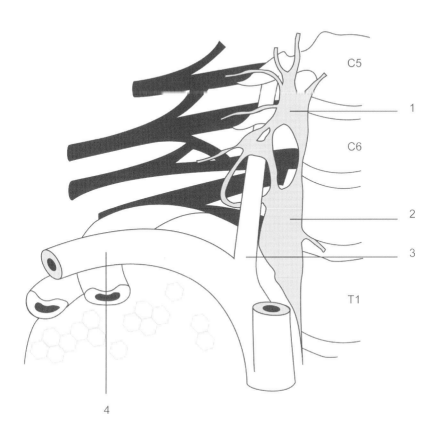

Figure 2.5 Stellate ganglion.
1. Middle cervical ganglion; 2. Stellate ganglion; 3. Vertebral artery; 4. Subclavian artery.

Examiner's mark sheet

marks

In Figure 2.5 identify the stellate ganglion and the   2   ☐
vertebral artery

At what vertebral level is the stellate ganglion   1   ☐
located?

C7-T1.

Describe the technique of blocking the stellate ganglion 5 ☐

- ◆ Preparation: ensures that the patient has been consented and all drugs and equipment are available and checked.
- ◆ Mentions aseptic precautions.
- ◆ Position: supine with neck extension.
- ◆ Point of insertion: between the trachea and carotid sheath at the level of the cricoid, and Chassaignac'c tubercle of C6 vertebra.
- ◆ Negative aspiration and injection of local anaesthetic.

If the stellate ganglion is at the level of C7 why are you aiming at the C6 tubercle? 2 ☐

- ◆ To avoid the lungs.
- ◆ To avoid the vertebral artery (that passes through the foramen transversarium at C6 level).

Give two indications for stellate ganglion block 2 ☐

Pain syndromes

Complex regional pain syndrome (CRPS) Type I and II, refractory angina and phantom limb pain.

Vascular insufficiency

Raynaud's syndrome, frostbite, obliterative vascular disease, vasospasm and emboli.

Give two features for a successful block 2 ☐

Horner's syndrome and an increase in temperature of the ipsilateral upper limb.

OSCE set 2

97

What are the features of Horner's syndrome?   2

Ptosis, miosis, anhydrosis, enophthalmos and loss of ciliospinal reflex.

Name four complications of stellate ganglion block   4

Needle in the wrong place

- Vascular injury: haematoma, trauma to carotid artery or the internal jugular vein (IJV).
- Neural injury: vagus, brachial plexus roots.
- Pulmonary injury: pneumothorax, haemothorax and chylothorax.
- Oesophageal perforation.

Spread of local anaesthetic

- Intravascular injection: carotid artery, vertebral artery and the IJV.
- Epidural block, intrathecal.
- Brachial plexus anaesthesia or injury (intraneural injection).
- Local spread: hoarseness (recurrent laryngeal nerve); elevated hemidiaphragm (phrenic nerve).

Infection

- Soft tissue (abscess), neuraxial (meningitis), bone (osteitis).

| Total: | /20 |

Technique of stellate ganglion block

The patient is placed in the supine position with the neck slightly extended and the head rotated slightly to the side opposite the block. The point of needle puncture is located between the trachea and the carotid sheath at the level of the cricoid cartilage and Chassaignac's tubercle - the anterior tubercle of the transverse process of C6.

The sternocleidomastoid and carotid artery are retracted laterally as the index and middle fingers palpate Chassaignac's tubercle. The skin and subcutaneous tissue are pressed firmly onto the tubercle to reduce the distance between the skin surface and bone, and in an attempt to push the dome of the lung out of the path of the needle. The needle is directed onto the tubercle, and then redirected medially and inferiorly towards the body of C6. After the body is contacted, the needle is withdrawn 1-2mm. This brings the needle out of the belly of the longus colli muscle, which sits posterior to the ganglion and runs along the anterolateral surface of the cervical vertebral bodies. The needle is then held immobile. The chosen local anaesthetic is slowly injected in small aliquots after careful negative aspiration. An initial 0.5cc test dose is given to rule out intravascular (vertebral artery) placement.

Key points

- The stellate ganglion is located at the level of C7-T1.
- It is blocked for pain conditions or vascular insufficiency.
- The anterior paratracheal route is used to approach the stellate ganglion.
- Successful stellate ganglion block is characterised by Horner's syndrome.
- Important risks include vertebral artery puncture, recurrent laryngeal nerve and phrenic nerve paralysis.

Station 2.6 Communication: brain stem test

Information for the candidate

A 20-year-old boy was admitted to ICU with a traumatic brain injury following a road traffic accident 48 hours ago. GCS at the scene was 5/15. He was intubated and ventilated by a paramedic and transferred to Accident and Emergency. A CT scan shows extensive cerebral contusions, massive haematoma and significant cerebral oedema. Both the neurosurgeons and intensivists have decided to do brain stem tests.

In this station you will be meeting the patient's father.

Examiner's mark sheet

marks

Introduces him/herself to the patient's relative.	1 ☐
Confirms that he/she is talking to the right person.	1 ☐
Asks the relative about the information already given by others (tell me what you know about his condition).	2 ☐
Explains that the patient has been on a breathing machine and breathing support.	2 ☐
Explains the scan findings.	2 ☐
Explains about the neurosurgical review and opinion.	2 ☐
Explains the procedure of a brain stem test.	3 ☐
The test will be repeated again before making any further decision.	2 ☐
Explains the significance of a brain stem test and switching off the breathing machine.	2 ☐
Attempts to find out the possibility of organ donation and to seek an advance directive.	2 ☐
Reassures appropriately that at all the above stages someone will come back and explain the results and decisions.	1 ☐

Total: /20

Information for the actor

Your son had a car accident 48 hours ago. All you know is that he has a severe head injury, his brain has been damaged and he has a big blood clot on the brain. He has been admitted to intensive care and is on life support with a breathing machine. You saw him last night and the nurse told you that his condition is very serious. You want to know more. You are hoping that he will recover.

You have been waiting to talk to the doctor to find out more details. You are devastated. Now, a doctor from the intensive care unit has come to talk to you.

General principles of communication

- Introduce and explain your role and the purpose of the interview.
- Establish the understanding and knowledge of the person about the given clinical scenario.
- Be honest and provide the correct information and facts.
- Explain in simple language, in words that are understandable to the patient and relatives.
- Listen actively to what the patient or relative is trying to express.
- Appropriate empathy or reassurance should be offered.
- Respond to verbal and non-verbal cues.
- Try to summarise and clarify, and provide an opportunity for further clarification.
- There should be a smooth conclusion without ending the interview abruptly.

Brain stem test

The brain stem test is done to confirm brain stem death. The three preconditions are:

- Apnoea and mechanically ventilated.
- An established cause for coma which can lead to irreversible brain injury.
- Exclusion of reversible causes.

Patient information

When the brain stem stops working, the brain cannot send messages to the body to control our unconscious functions, and equally cannot receive messages back from the body. If this is the case, then the person has no chance of recovery and according to UK law, the person has died.

The tests

A series of strict tests need to be carried out by two senior doctors at your son's bedside: his pupils do not respond to a direct light being shone in his eyes; his eyes do not blink when the surface of the eyeball is stroked with a piece of tissue or cotton wool; his natural eye movements are absent; and he does not breathe when taken off the ventilator. During this time, it is necessary for the level of CO_2 in his blood to rise and exceed the level required to stimulate a breath. He does not show any cough or gag reflex when the back of the throat is stimulated or the breathing tube is suctioned and he does not respond to pain when pressure is applied to certain areas of the body. These tests are frequently repeated to confirm that his brain stem has stopped working.

Why do you need to stop the painkillers and sleeping medicines?

These medications can have an effect on your son's reactions to these tests and so we must make sure that the effects of the medications have worn off completely before carrying out the tests.

Is the heart still beating?

The body's organs can continue to function for a short time while connected to a ventilator. However, if there is already brain stem death, this means that there is no chance of recovery.

Are these tests anything to do with organ donation?

No. It is usual practice to carry out these tests to confirm whether the brain stem has stopped working, regardless of any planned organ donation.

Key points

◆ The brain stem test involves a series of tests to confirm that the brain stem is not functioning.

◆ Confirmation of brain stem death means that death has occurred. It may be a difficult concept for the patient's relatives to understand.

◆ The patient's relatives may be subjected to psychological stress; therefore, appropriate support (presence of an ICU nurse) is important.

Station 2.7 Technical skill: lumbar puncture for spinal anaesthesia

Information for the candidate

In this station you will be asked to identify landmarks and describe the technique of performing spinal anaesthesia.

Examiner's mark sheet

marks

Indicate the space where you are going to perform the lumbar puncture (on an actor)   2 ☐

Identifica landmarks (iliac crests at L3/4 or L4 spinous process) with the patient sitting or in a lateral position.

The inter-space chosen must be no higher than L3/4.

Now describe how you would usually perform a spinal anaesthetic   10 ☐

◆ Ensures that the patient is consented and that resuscitation drugs and equipment are available.

◆ IV access must be obtained.

- Monitoring (ECG, NIBP, SpO$_2$).
- Ensures appropriate sterility (gown, gloves, cap and mask).
- Back preparation with antiseptic solution and sterile draping.
- Local anaesthetic is infiltrated.

Which of the following needles in Figure 2.7a would you prefer to use?

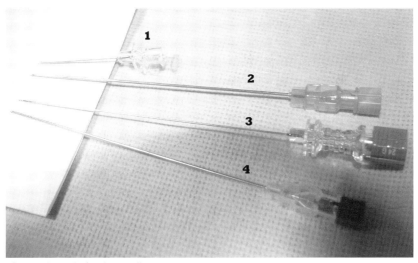

Figure 2.7a Spinal needles.
1. Introducer needle; 2. Whitacre needle; 3. Sprotte needle; 4. Quincke needle.

- A pencil-point needle smaller than 24 gauge is usually chosen.
- An introducer needle is inserted first into the interspace.
- A spinal needle is then introduced with loss of resistance when the dura is pierced.
- Free CSF flow should be observed.

What would you do if the fluid was blood-stained?   1 ☐

Wait until the CSF becomes clear and then inject; if it remains bloody, then re-site.

How much local anaesthetic would you use for each spinal segment to be blocked?

1 ☐

About 0.2ml per segment.

Name two factors affecting the spread of local anaesthetic in spinal anaesthesia

2 ☐

◆ Baricity of local anaesthetic injection.
◆ Position of the patient.

Give four contra-indications to performing spinal anaesthesia

4 ☐

◆ Patient refusal.
◆ Systemic or local infection.
◆ Abnormal clotting.
◆ Raised intracranial pressure.

| Total: | /20 |

Spinal anaesthesia

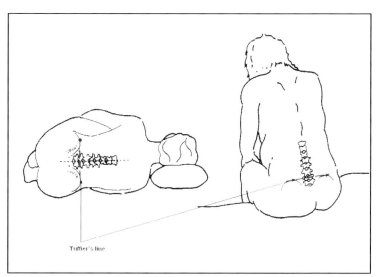

Tuffier's line

Figure 2.7b Landmarks for spinal anaesthesia.

The following steps should be performed for any nerve block or neuraxial block technique:

◆ Preparation of the patient: explain the procedure, describe the possible complications, and obtain consent.
◆ Preparation of the room. check the anaesthetic machine, have all resuscitation drugs and equipment ready, prepare the right amount of local anaesthetic, and have a trained assistant present. Secure intravenous access and institute appropriate monitors.
◆ Preparation of site: position correctly, ensure sterile precautions and perform the block.
◆ Post-procedure: monitor the vital parameters, maintain verbal contact with the patient and check the adequacy of the block.

The level of anaesthesia achieved depends on the volume of local anaesthetic injected and baricity of the solution, height of the patient and patient position. In an average 70Kg man, a volume of 1-1.5ml of 0.5% bupivacaine produces saddle block, 2-2.5ml produces a block to T10 and 2.5-3.0ml produces a block to T4-T6.

Blood supply to the spinal cord

The spinal cord receives its blood supply from one anterior and two posterior spinal arteries. The anterior spinal artery is formed at the level of the foramen magnum, by the joining of the branches of each vertebral artery. There are two posterior spinal arteries originating from postero-inferior cerebellar arteries. The posterior spinal arteries are supplemented by the spinal branches of the vertebral, deep cervical, intercostal, lumbar and the lateral sacral arteries.

The anterior spinal artery is joined by radicular arteries. Most of them are small, except one which is termed the arteria radicularis magna, or the artery of Adamkiewicz. It usually arises from the aorta in the lower thoracic or upper lumbar level. Damage to this artery can result in anterior spinal artery syndrome.

Key points

◆ A line drawn through most prominent points of the iliac crest passes through the spinous process of L4 or the L3-4 interspace.

◆ The procedure can be performed either in a sitting or a lateral position.

◆ Baricity, amount, patient positioning and height of the patient are known factors influencing the level of block.

◆ Use of pencil-point needles with a smaller size (less than 24 gauge) reduces the incidence of post-dural puncture headache.

Station 2.8 Clinical examination: cardiovascular system

Information for the candidate

In the following station you will be asked to examine the cardiovascular system of a patient who has presented for pre-operative assessment.

Examiner's mark sheet

marks

Introduces him/herself to the patient and explains his/her role. 1 ☐

Looks for clubbing. 1 ☐

Tongue: cyanosis. 1 ☐

Conjuctiva for pallor. 1 ☐

Looks for peripheral oedema/ankle oedema. 1 ☐

Pulses: examines the radial pulses, rate, rhythm, quality and character. 2 ☐

Compares the pulse on both sides.   1 ☐

Measures blood pressure.   2 ☐

Checks for jugular venous pressure (JVP).   2 ☐

Inspects chest.   1 ☐

Palpation of the chest

◆ Locates the apical impulse.   1 ☐

◆ Feels for thrills and para-sternal heave.   1 ☐

Auscultation of the chest

◆ All four areas in a systematic order.   2 ☐

◆ 1st and 2nd heart sounds.   1 ☐

◆ Auscultates the lung bases.   2 ☐

Total:	/20

Examination of the cardiovascular system

◆ Start with general appearance: posture, cachexia, breathlessness or distress.

◆ General examination: look for anaemia, icterus, cyanosis, clubbing and pedal oedema.

◆ Hands: patients with heart failure are vasoconstricted and their hands feel cold. Splinter haemorrhages are seen in infective endocarditis. Finger clubbing is seen in endocarditis and in cyanotic heart disease.

- Pulse: rate, rhythm, volume, character, radio-femoral delay, left/right asymmetry.
- The radial pulse is used to assess the rate and rhythm. In coarctation of the aorta, femoral pulses are weak and delayed, compared to the radial pulse (radiofemoral delay).
- Blood pressure is measured using the correct size of cuff, preferably on both arms.
- Check for a jugular venous pulse (for a method of checking this, refer to OSCE set 5, station 5.8).
- Inspection: face, neck, precordium, visible apical impulse, abnormal pulsations (supra-sternal, precordial, chest wall), back, abdomen.
- Palpation: apical impulse, parasternal heave and thrill.
- Apical impulse: palpate the precordium by laying the flat of the hand and outstretched fingers on the lower part of the chest wall to the left of the sternum. The apical impulse is located as the most outward and downward point at which pulsation is easily palpable. The normal position of the apex beat is the 5th intercostal space, medial to or at the midclavicular line.
- Auscultation: mitral, tricuspid, pulmonary and aortic areas for normal and additional heart sounds, and murmurs; lung bases for crepitations.

Key points

- Follow a methodical order of clinical examination: general examination, inspection, palpation and auscultation.
- Look for general features of cardiovascular disease.
- Elicit both normal and abnormal clinical signs.

Station 2.9 Measuring equipment: Wright respirometer

Information for the candidate

In this station you will be asked questions on equipment in order to assess your knowledge on measurement of volume and flow.

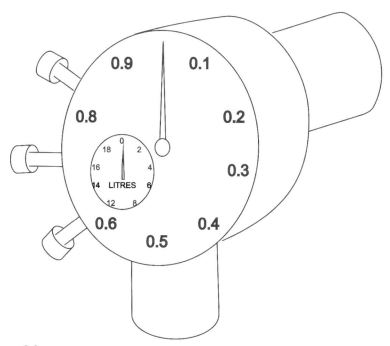

Figure 2.9.

Examiner's mark sheet

marks

Can you name this device? 1 ☐

Wright respirometer.

What does it measure?　2　☐

Tidal volume and minute volume.

What is the mechanism involved?　2　☐

It works by directing the breathing gases through oblique slots in a small cylinder enclosing a small vane which is made to rotate. The spindle on which the vane is mounted is connected to a pointer which moves over a dial indicating the volume of gas passed.

Can it be used to measure bidirectional flow?　1　☐

No. Gases that flow back through the device do not register since the flow in the reverse direction impinges on the bottom edge of the vane without producing any rotational movement.

What is the advantage of a Wright respirometer?　2　☐

It is a small, portable device used to measure tidal volume that does not require an electrical supply.

What are the disadvantages?　4　☐

- A minimum flow of 2L/minute is required.
- Over-reads at high flow, under-reads at low flow.
- Water condensation can cause the pointer to stick.
- No display of measured volume (no electrical output).

What is the resistance to breathing through this?　2　☐

It is low and is about $2cmH_2O$ at 100L/minute.

Can you name two devices to measure flow?　2　☐

- Pneumotachograph (constant orifice, variable pressure).
- Rotameter (constant pressure, variable orifice).

What is the principle behind a pneumotachograph?   2 ☐

A pneumotachograph is a constant orifice variable pressure flow meter. As the gas flows through the fixed resistance there will be a drop in pressure. A differential pressure transducer senses the pressure gradient across the resistance. The change in pressure is proportional to the flow.

What are the advantages of a pneumotachograph?   2 ☐

High accuracy and the ability to display the readings.

Total:	/20

Measurement of volume and flow

The Wright respirometer is a simple device used to measure the tidal volume. On the outer surface of the case there are on/off and reset buttons. Due to inertia it under-reads at low flows and because of momentum it over-reads at high flows. It has two display dials. The outer one is calibrated at 100ml per division and a smaller inner display is calibrated at 1L per division. Water condensation from expired moisture can prevent the free rotation of the vane. It does not have any alarms. In recent versions the flow can be detected electronically which will be more accurate at low flows.

Gas volume can be measured directly using a gas meter, vitalograph and water displacement spirometer (Benedict-Roth wet spirometer).

Gas volume can be measured indirectly by measuring the pressure drop across a resistance, by measuring the heat transfer or by measuring the mechanical movement resulting from kinetic energy of gas flow. In the rotameter and peak flow meter, the orifice through which gas flows enlarges with increasing flow rate and the pressure drop across the orifice remains constant.

A pneumotachograph is a constant orifice variable pressure drop flow meter. The pressure drop in this device is also influenced by gas composition, temperature and viscosity. The device is designed to measure laminar flow. The values can change in turbulent flow.

Key points

- The Wright respirometer is a simple, portable device used for gas volume measurement.
- It measures flow in only one direction.
- It over-reads at high flows and under-reads at low flows.

Station 2.10 Resuscitation: basic life support of a pregnant mother

Information for the candidate

You are the resident anaesthetist on call and have been bleeped to urgently attend a 36-week pregnant woman who has collapsed on the labour ward.

Examiner's mark sheet

marks

Ensures safety of the patient and self (safe to approach) and checks for responsiveness (no response).   2 ☐

Confirms cardiorespiratory arrest: 2 ☐

- Looks/listens/feels for breath after manoeuvres to open the airway.
- Palpates the carotid pulse.

(Both manoeuvres to be done simultaneously for 10 seconds).

Calls for help (specifies obstetrician and paediatrician in addition to the crash team).   2 ☐

Relieves aorto-caval compression (wedge under right buttock or manual displacement of the uterus or a left lateral tilt).   2 ☐

Commences CPR (bag and mask available).   2 ☐
Compression: ventilation ratio 30:2 (100 compressions/minute).

Help arrives. She has started making some attempts to breathe. On connecting her to the monitor, the ECG rhythm shows bradycardia with a heart rate of 38/minute. How would you manage this patient?   4 ☐

Look for adverse signs: rate <40 beats per minute, BP <90 mmHg systolic, heart failure, ventricular arrhythmias.

How would you treat this patient?   2 ☐

By administering intravenous atropine 500µg.

What is the maximum recommended dose of atropine?   1 ☐

Maximum of 3mg atropine in aliquots of 500µg.

What factors would suggest a risk of asystole?   3 ☐

Recent asystole, Mobitz Type 2 block, complete heart block with a broad QRS or a ventricular pause of more than 3 seconds.

Total: /20

Cardiopulmonary resuscitation in pregnancy

The physiological changes during pregnancy can cause additional problems during resuscitation. Cardiac output, blood volume and oxygen consumption all increase during pregnancy. The fetus should always be considered when a cardiac arrest occurs in pregnant women. The gravid uterus may cause significant compression of the iliac and abdominal vessels, reducing venous return from the lower limbs, resulting in reduced cardiac output. Important causes of maternal death include thrombo-embolism, a hypertensive disorder of pregnancy, haemorrhage, amniotic fluid embolism and pre-existing cardiac disease.

There is an increased risk of acid aspiration in pregnancy; therefore, the correct application of cricoid pressure and early tracheal intubation to protect the lungs are important. Tracheal intubation may be more difficult in the pregnant patient, due to anatomical changes in the upper airway. Ectopic pregnancy, placental abruption and uterine rupture can lead to massive haemorrhage in pregnancy.

If immediate resuscitation attempts fail, an emergency Caesarean section should be considered. There are better chances of an infant's survival if the emergency Caesarean section is done within 5 minutes of cardiac arrest.

Key points

- The obstetrician and neonatologist should be involved at an early stage.
- The principles of adult basic and advanced life support apply to pregnant patients as well.
- Early tracheal intubation, along with cricoid pressure, can reduce the risk of aspiration.
- The importance of manoeuvres to relieve aorto-caval compression cannot be over-emphasized.
- Emergency Caesarean section is indicated to improve the chances of both maternal and fetal survival, if resuscitation is unsuccessful after 5 minutes.

Station 2.11 Anatomy: vagus nerve

Information for the candidate

In this station you will be asked questions on anatomy of one of the cranial nerves which is of special interest to anaesthetists.

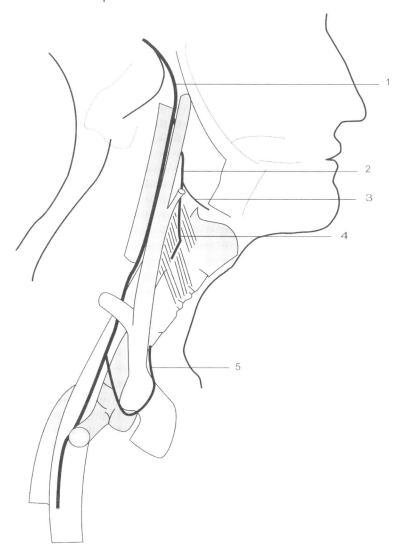

Figure 2.11 Course and distribution of the vagus nerve.

Examiner's mark sheet

marks

Name the structures labelled 1-4 in Figure 2.11   4 ☐

1. Vagus nerve.
2. Superior laryngeal nerve.
3. Internal laryngeal nerve.
4. External laryngeal nerve.
5. Recurrent laryngeal nerve.

What is the origin of the vagus nerve?   1 ☐

It originates from the medulla oblongata.

How many nuclei does it have and what are they?   3 ☐

Three. They are:

◆   Dorsal nucleus.
◆   Nucleus ambiguus.
◆   Nucleus tractus solitarius.

Through which foramen does it leave the skull?   1 ☐

Jugular foramen.

Name two other structures that pass through this foramen   2 ☐

Accessory nerve, glossopharyngeal nerve, internal jugular vein (IJV).

State the relations of the vagus nerve in the neck   2 ☐

In the neck, it passes down within the carotid sheath, lying between the IJV and internal carotid artery. Beyond the level of the upper border of the thyroid cartilage it lies between the IJV and common carotid artery.

What is the course of the right vagus nerve inside the thorax?

2 ▢

On the right side, the nerve passes across the subclavian artery between it and the right innominate vein and descends by the side of the trachea to the back of the root of the lung where it spreads out in the posterior pulmonary plexus. From the lower part of this plexus two cords descend on the oesophagus, and divide to form, with branches from the opposite nerve, the oesophageal plexus.

What is the course of the left vagus nerve inside the thorax?

2 ▢

On the left side, the vagus enters the thorax between the left carotid and subclavian arteries, behind the left innominate vein. It crosses the left side of the arch of the aorta, and descends behind the root of the left lung, forming the posterior pulmonary plexus. From this it runs along the anterior surface of the oesophagus, where it unites with the nerve of the right side in the oesophageal plexus.

Apart from the laryngeal branches can you name three other branches of the vagus nerve?

3 ▢

- In the jugular foramen: meningeal and auricular.
- In the neck: pharyngeal (superior laryngeal nerve, recurrent laryngeal, superior cardiac).
- In the thorax: inferior cardiac, anterior and posterior bronchial, oesophageal.
- In the abdomen: gastric, coeliac, hepatic.

| Total: | /20 |

Key points

- The vagus is the largest and most widely distributed cranial nerve.
- It arises as a group of rootlets on the anterolateral surface of the medulla oblongata. After crossing the posterior cranial fossa it leaves the skull through the jugular foramen.
- The right vagus nerve enters the thorax between the innominate vein and subclavian artery. The left vagus nerve enters the thorax behind the left innominate vein.

Station 2.12 History taking: laparoscopic cholecystectomy

Information for the candidate

In this station you will be asked to take a history from a 40-year-old female patient presenting for a laparoscopic cholecystectomy.

Examiner's mark sheet

	marks	
Introduces him/herself to the patient.	1	☐
Confirms that he/she is talking to the right person and the proposed surgery.	1	☐
H/O previous operations; Caesarean section under GA, arthroscopy.	2	☐
H/O awareness during Caesarean section.	1	☐
Type of awareness: conscious recall, unpleasant dreams, etc.	2	☐
Asks about further details on pain experienced during awareness and counselling received or offered.	2	☐

Hospital admission with cholecystitis 6 months ago.	2	☐
H/O heartburn but no reflux.	2	☐
H/O hypertension.	1	☐
Blood pressure well controlled with amlodipine.	2	☐
H/O smoking: does not smoke.	1	☐
H/O alcohol intake: a glass of wine every night.	1	☐
H/O allergy: no known allergy.	2	☐

Total:	/20

Information for the actor

You are scheduled to have an operation tomorrow (removal of the gallbladder through key-hole surgery). Six months ago you were in hospital with tummy pain and you also felt very sick during that time. You never had jaundice. You do not smoke but take a glass of wine every night. You had an ultrasound scan of your tummy which showed you have gallstones. You also had a camera put down your throat into the food pipe and the result was normal. The treatment for gallstones is removal of the gallbladder.

You are taking medicine for high blood pressure (amlodipine 10mg tablet every night). You also have a high cholesterol and you are on a medicine, simvastatin. You had two operations in the past: Caesarean section, 10 years ago, during which you remember a tube going down your throat and somebody pressing on your throat while going to sleep. You have seen a specialist and you understand the reason why you remember this, so you are not too concerned about that now. Your Caesarean section was an emergency operation and you probably had a low dose of anaesthetic so that the anaesthetic would not affect the baby. Since then you have had an

Ensures that the head and neck position is optimal (sniffing the   2   ☐
morning air position, extension at the atlanto-occipital joint and
flexion of the neck).

Releases or reduces the cricoid pressure transiently and   2   ☐
reapplies if no improvement.

Attempts an optimum external laryngeal manoeuvre, which   2   ☐
includes backward, upward and right-ward pressure (BURP)
on the thyroid cartilage.

Still it is a grade 3 view

Calls for help.   2   ☐

Requests an alternative laryngoscope blade or McCoy   2   ☐
laryngoscope.

Requests a gum elastic bougie.   2   ☐

Oxygen saturation decreases to 90% and the low saturation alarm sounds

Ventilates with a bag and mask with 100% oxygen, continues   2   ☐
cricoid pressure and wakes up the patient.

Total:	/20

Information for the examiner

The patient has been pre-oxygenated for 3 minutes and has just received thiopentone and suxamethonium. Please hand over the case to the candidate soon after administering the thiopentone and suxamethonium. Set the airway parameters of SimMan to a grade 3 view of the larynx by selecting neck stiffness and pharyngeal oedema.

Failed intubation scenario

Cricothyrotomy should be performed to oxygenate the patient if this scenario progresses to a 'cannot intubate, cannot ventilate' (CICV) situation. A cricothyrotomy device (Quick trach or a jet ventilation cannula and a manual jet ventilator) should be requested immediately.

The basic plan for an unanticipated difficult intubation is as follows:

- ◆ A: initial tracheal intubation plan.
- ◆ B: secondary tracheal intubation plan, when plan A has failed.
- ◆ C: maintenance of oxygenation and ventilation, postponement of surgery and waking the patient when earlier plans fail.
- ◆ D: rescue techniques for a CICV scenario.

During initial tracheal intubation, an alternate laryngoscope, optimum head neck position and a BURP manoeuvre should be considered. A secondary tracheal intubation plan involves fibreoptic-assisted intubation through the laryngeal mask airway (LMA) and intubating the LMA.

Cricoid pressure can impair insertion of the laryngoscope, passage of an introducer and can cause airway obstruction. Cricoid pressure should be applied with an initial force of 10 N when the patient is awake, increasing to 30 N as consciousness is lost. The force should be reduced with suction at hand, if it impedes laryngoscopy or causes airway obstruction (refer to OSCE set 4, station 4.19).

Key points

- ◆ Effective airway management requires a careful primary plan with an adequate back-up plan when the primary plan fails.
- ◆ Maintenance of oxygenation takes priority over everything else during the execution of each plan.
- ◆ Seek the best assistance available as soon as difficulty with laryngoscopy is experienced
- ◆ In the given scenario in this station, there is an increased likelihood of regurgitation and pulmonary aspiration. Pre-oxygenation and cricoid pressure are very important.

- If intubation fails, despite a maximum of 3 attempts (including attempts with introducer and alternate blades), a failed intubation plan with the aim of maintaining oxygenation and waking the patient is initiated immediately.
- A further dose of suxamethonium should not be given.
- Based on the urgency of the surgical procedure, plan C varies. In general, appendicectomy can be delayed and so aim to wake the patient.
- Maintenance of ventilation and oxygenation is possible with a conventional bag and face mask, with or without an oral or nasal airway. If unsatisfactory, the LMA should be used. The Proseal LMA provides improved protection against aspiration.
- If ventilation is impossible and hypoxaemia develops, rescue techniques for the CICV situation, such as needle cricothryrotomy with transtracheal jet ventilation (TTJV), are implemented.

Station 2.14 Monitoring equipment: peripheral nerve stimulator

Information for the candidate

In this station your knowledge on equipment used for monitoring during anaesthesia will be tested.

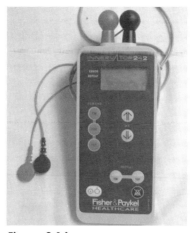

Figure 2.14a.

Examiner's mark sheet

marks

What is this equipment and what is its clinical use?   2 ☐

This is a peripheral nerve stimulator used to monitor neuromuscular function. At induction it is used to assess the depth of neuromuscular block, during the maintenance phase of anaesthesia to titrate the repeat dose of muscle relaxant and at recovery to assess the adequacy of reversal from neuromuscular block.

Name two factors which determine the energy requirement to propagate a nerve impulse   2 ☐

- Stimulus strength (current in mA).
- Duration of stimulus (milli seconds).

Why would you use a supramaximal stimulus?   1 ☐

To ensure all motor fibres of the nerve are stimulated.

Indicate where you would place the electrodes for stimulating the ulnar nerve   1 ☐

- Distal electrode: 1cm proximal to the flexion crease of the wrist.
- Proximal electrode: 2-3cm proximal to the distal electrode.

Indicate how you would connect the leads   2 ☐

Negative lead distally (negative on the nerve) and positive lead proximally.

Which muscle contraction would you observe when the ulnar nerve is stimulated?   1 ☐

Adductor pollicis brevis (adduction of thumb).

State three methods available to assess muscle contraction   3 ☐

◆ Visual.
◆ Tactile.
◆ Electromyography.
◆ Accelerography.
◆ Mechanomyography.

What is double-burst stimulation (DBS)?   2 ☐

DBS consists of two short bursts of 50-Hz tetanic stimulation separated by 750ms.

What is a post-tetanic count (PTC)?   2 ☐

Single-twitch stimulations following a tetanic stimulation and count the responses.

What is the mechanism behind a post-tetanic count?   2 ☐

Tetanic stimulation increases mobilisation of acetylcholine (Ach). Subsequent single twitches release a supranormal concentration of Ach.

What is the significance of a post-tetanic count?   2 ☐

PTC <5: profound block; >15 equal to two twitches of train of four (TOF).

Total: /20

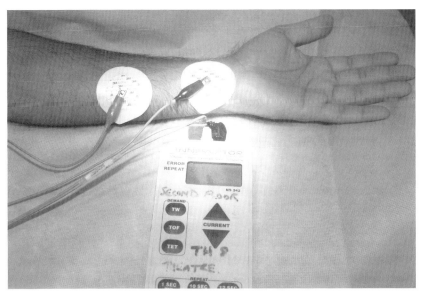

Figure 2.14b Placement of electrodes for ulnar nerve stimulation.

Neuromuscular monitoring

Factors determining the response to the nerve stimulation are:

- Stimulus strength: the rheobase is the minimal current required to create a nerve impulse.
- Duration of the stimulus: the chronaxie is the duration of the stimulus required to stimulate at twice the rheobase.

Supramaximal stimulation

The reaction of a single muscle fibre to an electrical stimulus follows an all-or-none law. Each fibre of a muscle will either contract maximally or will not contract at all. This means that a strong enough stimulus impulse (maximal stimulus) is required for all fibres of the stimulated muscle to contract. Increasing the stimulus above the maximal level does not produce a stronger response. A current setting of 60mA will achieve supramaximal stimulation in most cases.

Places the paddles back on the defibrillator.   2 ☐

**How would you place the paddles if someone has a   2 ☐
pacemaker?**

The defibrillator electrodes should be placed at least 12-15cm
from the pacemaker unit.

**What do these symbols in Figures 2.15a and 2.15b   2 ☐
indicate?**

Figure 2.15a.

Figure 2.15b.

Figure 2.15a shows a Type BF defibrillation proof equipment. Figure 2.15b shows a Type CF defibrillation proof equipment.

Total: /20

Safe use of the defibrillator

Confirm the diagnosis of VF to avoid the inappropriate delivery of shock. Check the connection of leads. Adult paddles have a typical diameter of 13cm. Conductive gel pads improve electrical contact between the paddles and chest. A firm pressure of 10Kg force is used.

The standard procedure is to place one electrode to the right of the upper sternum below the clavicle and the other level with the 5th left intercostal space in the anterior axillary line. It allows maximum current flow through the myocardium. If the patient has a cardiac pacemaker, the current may travel along the pacemaker wire causing burns where the electrode tip makes contact with the myocardium. Placing the defibrillator electrodes at least 12-15cm from the pacemaker unit should minimise the risk. Antero-posterior electrode placement can also be used in patents with a pacemaker. The anterior electrode is placed on the left anterior chest, midway between the xiphoid process and left nipple, corresponding to the V2-V3 ECG electrode position. The posterior electrode should be placed beneath the left scapula.

The paddles should either be on the equipment or on the patient's chest. It should be charged only when on the patient's chest. A charged paddle in the air can cause arcing and accident.

If the defibrillator is charged but a shock is no longer indicated, it should be discharged through the defibrillator internally (by altering the energy ootting) before removing the paddles from the chest.

Since you sustained the head injury you suffer from fitting, but for the last 2 years you have had no fits.

You quit smoking 2 weeks ago and you don't drink alcohol. You regularly take phenytoin tablets for fits and the contraceptive pill, and are allergic to nuts; they give you a rash and your face swells.

Key points

◆ Follow a structured approach.
◆ Enquire as to all the details of past medical history.
◆ Elicit the nature and severity of any drug allergy.

(For more information please refer to OSCE set 1, station 1.12).

Station 2.18 Communication: suxamethonium apnoea

Information for the candidate

As the on-call anaesthetist, you have just given an anaesthetic to a fit and well 10-year-old girl for an urgent appendicectomy. General anaesthesia was induced with a rapid sequence technique using thiopentone and suxamethonium. At the end of the surgery, the child would not breathe. She is haemodynamically stable. Her HR is 80 bpm, BP is 100/60 mm Hg, SpO_2 is 100%, $EtCO_2$ is 5.5 kPa, tympanic temperature is 36.8°C, and her pupils are midsize and reacting. Neuromuscular monitoring with train of four is suggestive of suxamethonium apnoea. The child is now sedated and ventilated in intensive care.

In this station you will meet the mother of the child.

Examiner's mark sheet

marks

Introduces him/herself to the patient's relative.   1 ☐

Confirms that he/she is talking to the right person.   1 ☐

Clearly explains the reason for admitting to intensive care.   2 ☐

Avoids jargon.   1 ☐

Reassures that her daughter is sedated (kept sleepy), pain-free and should wake up in 4-6 hours time.   2 ☐

Explains that suxamethonium was the correct drug to use and why it was used.   2 ☐

Mentions that this is a recognised complication of suxamethonium.   1 ☐

Explains the reason why her daughter is not able to breathe after suxamethonium.   2 ☐

Explains blood tests for suxamethonium apnoea.   2 ☐

Explains that her daughter can safely have anaesthetics in the future.   1 ☐

Confirms he/she will write to the general practitioner.   2 ☐

Emphasises the need for the entire family to undergo a blood test for suxamethonium apnoea.   2 ☐

Sympathetic throughout and satisfactory conclusion.   1 ☐

Total: /20

the nerve passes behind and across the posterior aspect of the humerus. It runs between the medial and long heads of triceps and supplies the triceps muscle. It also gives rise to sensory branches to the posterior aspect of the arm. Further down its course, between the lateral epicondyle (of the humerus) and musculospiral groove, the nerve divides into 2 terminal branches: superficial and deep. The deep branch supplies the extensor muscles of the forearm. The superficial branch courses along with the radial artery and provides sensory innervation to the dorsal aspect of the wrist and thumb, and the index and middle fingers.

At the level of the elbow, with all aseptic precautions, the nerve is blocked at the level of the crease or 1-2cm above the crease line. The short bevel needle is inserted just lateral to the biceps tendon, between the biceps tendon and brachioradialis muscle. Although conventionally paraesthesia was elicited to confirm vicinity to the nerve, a nerve stimulator can easily be used to increase success rate. The motor response to stimulation is extension of the wrist and fingers. Recently, ultrasound-guided blocks have gained popularity.

Median nerve block at the elbow

The median nerve is made up of fibres from C5-T1. In the axilla, the nerve lies anterior and superior to the axillary artery. After leaving the axilla, the nerve closely follows the course of the brachial artery. At the level of the elbow the median nerve lies medial to the brachial artery which in turn lies medial to the tendon of biceps. Further down, the nerve provides motor innervation to the flexor muscles of the forearm. As the nerve approaches the wrist it lies deep to and between the tendons of the palmaris longus and flexor carpi radialis muscles.

At the level of the elbow, the nerve is blocked at the crease level. Using a 1½-inch short bevelled needle the nerve is located medial to brachial artery pulsation. The nerve is located using paraesthesia, a nerve stimulator or ultrasound-guided techniques. When stimulated at this level the motor response would include flexion of the wrist and abduction of the thumb.

Ulnar nerve block at the elbow

The ulnar nerve is made up of fibres from C6-T1. The nerve lies anterior and inferior to the axillary artery in the axilla. It initially follows the brachial artery and later courses medially to pass between the olecranon process and medial opicondyle of the humerus. The nerve courses down between the two heads of flexor carpi ulnaris muscle and then moves along with the ulnar artery. About 2cm proximal to the wrist crease, the nerve divides into dorsal and palmar branches.

At the level of the elbow, posteriorly, the olecranon process (the proximal bony process of the ulna that fits into the olecranon fossa of the humerus) and the medial epicondyle of the humerus are identified. The ulnar sulcus between these 2 bony landmarks is palpated. Under aseptic precautions the short bevelled needle is inserted just proximal to the sulcus in a slight cephalad trajectory. The nerve is fairly superficial in this location.

Use of a peripheral nerve stimulator for nerve blocks

Stimulation of nerves with low intensity current is used to locate the nerves. It requires a nerve stimulator able to deliver low intensity current and an insulated needle with an electrical lead attachment. Initial output of 1-1.5mA is usually chosen. A frequency of 2Hz is used. Higher frequency causes tetanic stimulation; lower frequency can miss the nerve. Once the motor response is elicited, current output is reduced and the threshold at which twitches disappear is noted. Strong twitches elicited at a low intensity of current (e.g. <0.2 mA) may suggest intra-neural placement of the needle.

Key points

♦ The median nerve lies medial to brachial artery pulsation.
♦ The ulnar nerve should be blocked 2-3cm proximal to the medial epicondyle. The incidence of neuritis is high if blocked at the ulnar groove.
♦ The radial nerve is blocked between biceps tendon and brachioradialis.
♦ The peripheral nerve stimulator is useful to locate median, radial and ulnar nerves at the elbow.

Station 2.20 Technical skill: ankle block

Information for the candidate

A 60-year-old male patient is scheduled for a correction of hallux valgus of the left foot under regional block. Correction of hallux valgus involves an osteotomy and k-wire insertion at the first metatarsophalangeal joint.

Examiner's mark sheet

marks

Name the nerves that need to be blocked in order to provide anaesthesia for this surgical procedure   3 ☐

The three nerves that need to be blocked are:

- ◆ Superficial peroneal nerve.
- ◆ Deep peroneal (anterior tibial) nerve.
- ◆ Saphenous nerve.

What are the other two nerves in the ankle that are required to be blocked for a complete ankle block?   1 ☐

Tibial nerve and sural nerve.

Of the five nerves which one is not a branch of the sciatic nerve?   1 ☐

Saphenous nerve.

Name the structures labelled 1-5 in Figure 2.20   5 ☐

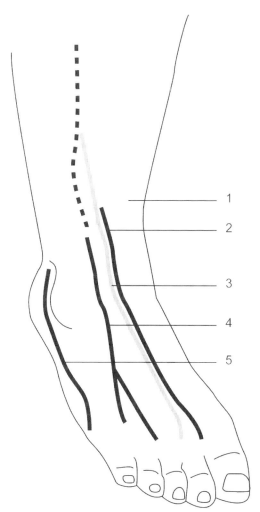

Figure 2.20 Nerve supply of the foot.

1. Extensor hallucis longus tendon.
2. Deep peroneal (anterior tibial) nerve.
3. Dorsalis pedis artery.
4. Superficial peroneal nerve.
5. Sural nerve.

Name the terminal branches of the tibial nerve   2 ☐

The tibial nerve divides into the medial and lateral plantar nerves.

How would you block the tibial nerve at the ankle?   2 ☐

The tibial nerve is blocked by injecting local anaesthetic behind the medial malleolus and anterior to the tibial artery pulsation.

How would you block the deep peroneal nerve?   2 ☐

It lies on the medial side of the dorsalis pedis artery. The nerve is blocked by injecting local anaesthetic on the medial side of the artery, between the artery and extensor hallucis longus (in the 1st metatarsal space).

Where would you inject local anaesthetic to block the sural nerve?   2 ☐

The sural nerve can be blocked by subcutaneous infiltration of local anaesthetic behind the lateral malleolus.

Where would you inject local anaesthetic to block the saphenous nerve?   2 ☐

Subcutaneous infiltration 5-10cm above the medial malleolus along the course of the long saphenous vein.

Total:	/20

Nerves of the leg

The sciatic nerve terminates in the apex of the popliteal fossa to divide into the common peroneal and tibial nerves. The tibial nerve leaves the popliteal fossa between the heads of gastrocnemius to run on the tibialis posterior, then passes medially and enters the foot behind the medial malleolus between the posterior tibial artery and flexor hallucis longus tendon. It terminates into the medial and lateral plantar branches which provide sensory supply to the sole of the foot.

In the popliteal fossa, the tibial nerve gives off a sensory branch, the sural nerve, which passes downwards along the lateral aspect of the leg and then behind the lateral malleolus to supply the foot.

The common peroneal nerve winds round the neck of the fibula and divides into superficial peroneal and deep peroneal branches. It is at this location that the nerve is vulnerable to pressure neuropathy. The superficial peroneal nerve provides sensory supply to the lower and outer aspect of the leg and dorsum of the foot. The deep peroneal nerve supplies the skin over the web space between the first and second toe.

Tibial nerve block at the ankle

The tibial nerve provides sensory innervation to the posterior portion of the calf, the heel, and the medial plantar surface. In the ankle, the nerve courses medially between the Achilles tendon and the medial malleolus, where it divides into the medial and lateral plantar nerves. To block the nerve, the area between the medial malleolus and the Achilles tendon is prepared. The nerve lies in the posterior groove of the medial malleolus and is blocked by inserting the short bevelled needle anterior to the posterior tibial artery pulsation.

Sural nerve block at the ankle

The sural nerve is a branch of the (posterior) tibial nerve. The nerve passes from the posterior calf around the lateral malleolus to provide sensory innervation of the posterolateral aspect of the calf, the plantar surface of heel, the lateral surface of the foot and the fifth toe. To block this nerve, the posterior groove behind the lateral malleolus is identified. The area between the lateral malleolus and Achilles tendon is prepared. The nerve is blocked either by eliciting paraesthesia in the groove or by subcutaneous infiltration behind the lateral malleolus.

Flow meters   3 ☐

◆ Checks all three valves are operational (O_2, N_2O, air).
◆ Checks for anti-hypoxia device (mention it).
◆ Checks for emergency oxygen flush.

Checks the vaporisers   4 ☐

◆ Adequately filled.
◆ Correctly seated.
◆ Checks for leak (both in the on and off position).
◆ Turns the vaporiser off when checks are completed.

What precautions would you take before fitting a   3 ☐
cylinder to the machine?

◆ Plastic dust cover is removed.
◆ Make sure the sealing washer is present.
◆ Before fitting, gently open the cylinder to let some gas escape.

Why would you do this?   1 ☐

To blow out any dust/grit from the outlet that might damage the pressure regulator.

Total:	/20

Anaesthesia machine check

In this OSCE station you are asked to check the anaesthetic machine. You have only 5 minutes to complete the task. It is vital that you follow a systematic order to identify any faults with the machine or monitoring equipment.

Check that the anaesthetic machine is connected to the electricity supply (if appropriate) and switched on

- Take note of any information or labelling on the anaesthetic machine referring to the current status of the machine. Servicing labels should be filed in the service logbook

Check that all monitoring devices, in particular the oxygen analyser, pulse oximeter, and capnograph are functioning and have appropriate alarm limits

- Check that gas sampling lines are properly attached and free of obstructions.
- Check that an appropriate frequency of recording non-invasive blood pressure is selected.

Check with a 'tug test' that each pipeline is correctly inserted into the appropriate gas supply terminal

- Ensure that an adequate supply of oxygen is available from a reserve oxygen cylinder.
- Check that adequate supplies of other gases (nitrous oxide, air) are available and connected as appropriate.
- Check the cylinder yoke; an empty yoke should be fitted with a blanking plug.
- Check that all pipeline pressure gauges in use on the anaesthetic machine indicate 400-500kPa.

Check the operation of flow meters

- Check that each flow valve operates smoothly and that the bobbin moves freely throughout its range.
- Check the anti-hypoxia device is working correctly.
- Check the operation of the emergency oxygen bypass control.

Check the vaporiser(s)

- Check that each vaporiser is adequately filled.
- Check that each vaporiser is correctly seated on the back bar and is not tilted.

Station 3.3 Data interpretation: ECG

Information for the candidate

In this station you will need to interpret the ECG of an elderly patient with a history of breathlessness in the past, now presenting for elective surgery.

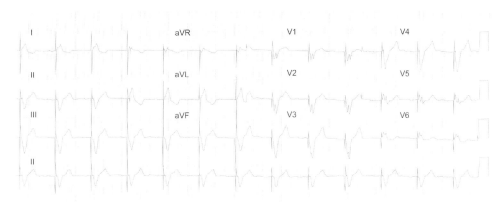

Figure 3.3 ECG.

Examiner's mark sheet

Please tick the correct answer - true or false.   *marks*

1. The standard speed of recording is 25mm/second.   True False 2 ☐
2. Standard calibration is 1mV = 1cm.   True False 2 ☐
3. The rhythm is sinus.   True False 2 ☐
4. The rate is 100 beats/minute.   True False 2 ☐
5. Left axis deviation is present.   True False 2 ☐
6. The PR interval is within the normal range.   True False 2 ☐
7. The QRS complex is widened.   True False 2 ☐

8. There is a left bundle branch block.   True   False   2 ☐
9. T waves are of normal morphology in all the leads.   True   False   2 ☐
10. The rhythm is suggestive of atrial pacing.   True   False   2 ☐

Total: /20

Answers

1. True.

2. True. Calibration is 1mV =10mm =1cm.

3. False. Pacemaker rhythm.

4. False. 75/minute.

5. True. There is a positive QRS in I and a negative QRS in III and aVF; common in the presence of a pacemaker.

6. False. The P wave is not seen and the pacemaker spike is followed by a QRS complex.

7. True. There is a widened QRS complex.

8. True. It is commonly present with a pacing rhythm.

9. False. Inverted T waves in I and aVL.

10. False. There are no P waves; it is suggestive of ventricular pacing.

Pacemakers

When the electrical activity of the heart is deranged either due to initiation of impulse (e.g. sinus node disorder, severe bradycardia) or due to failure of conduction of impulse (e.g. complete heart block, symptomatic trifascicular block), the mechanical activity of the heart fails, thereby reducing cardiac output. A pacemaker is a device to regulate the electrical activity of the heart.

Anatomy relevant to tracheostomy

In the adult, the epiglottis is at the level of C2, the vocal cord is at C4 and the cricoid is at C6. Anterior to the trachea lies the skin, subcutaneous tissue and strap muscles. The isthmus of the thyroid gland crosses the trachea over the second and third tracheal rings. The trachea is formed of semicircular cartilaginous rings anteriorly and laterally. The posterior aspect of the trachea and the spaces between the rings are membranous.

The brachiocephalic trunk crosses from left to right anterior to the trachea at the superior thoracic inlet behind the sternum. Abnormal anatomy of this artery or an aneurysm of the arch of the aorta can pose a life-threatening risk of bleeding if missed during examination prior to tracheostomy. Occasionally, the isthmus of the thyroid is supplied also by the thyroidea ima artery, a branch of the brachiocephalic trunk, the arch of the aorta or the left common carotid artery.

On the left side of the neck the thoracic duct forms an arch about 3-4cm above the clavicle. The vagus nerve, left common carotid artery and internal jugular vein lie anterior to the thoracic duct. The thoracic duct ends by opening into the junction of the left internal jugular vein and subclavian vein.

In adults the trachea is about 10cm long, extending from the larynx to the carina. It commences at the level of the C6 vertebra. The bifurcation of the trachea into main bronchi is located at the level of T4/T5. It comprises 15-20 U-shaped rings; posteriorly the gap is filled with a fibrous membrane.

The inferior thyroid vein (along with the recurrent laryngeal nerve) travels in the tracheo-oesophageal groove. The anterior jugular vein is formed by the confluence of several superficial veins from the submaxillary region. It descends between the anterior border of the sternocleidomastoid muscle and the midline of the neck. Just above the sternum the two anterior jugular veins communicate by a transverse trunk, the venous jugular arch, which receives tributaries from the inferior thyroid veins.

The carotid artery and internal jugular vein run laterally. These structures are vulnerable to injury during tracheostomy if the dissection goes lateral and deep.

Complications of tracheostomy

◆ Immediate complications include: bleeding, air embolism, subcutaneous emphysema, tracheostomy tube dislodgement.
◆ Delayed complications include: infection, mediastinal sepsis and tube blockage.
◆ Late complications include: tracheal stenosis and tracheocutaneous fistula.

Key points

◆ In the adult the cricoid cartilage is located at the level of the 6th cervical vertebra.
◆ At the level of the thoracic inlet there are highly vascular structures that lie anterior to the trachea.
◆ The trachea bifurcates into the main bronchi at the level of T4/T5.

Station 3.6 Communication: postponed surgery

Information for the candidate

In this station you will meet a patient who is scheduled for biopsy of a lesion inside the cheek of the mouth. She has to be cancelled today, because the list is over-running; the previous patient on the list haemorrhaged in the recovery room following radical neck dissection and was taken back to theatre, hence the delay.

Examiner's mark sheet

marks

Introduces him/herself and confirms that he/she is talking to the right person.   2

Palpation

Confirm the position of the trachea, symmetry of chest expansion (anterior and posterior), areas of tenderness or deformity, and tactile vocal fremitus (by asking the patient to say one, one ... or ninety-nine ...).

Percussion

Percuss for normal resonance, hyper-resonance (pneumothorax, large bulla, emphysema), dullness (consolidation, pleural effusion), and diaphragmatic excursion (find the level of diaphragmatic dullness on both sides. Ask the patient to take a deep breath; the level of dullness should move down by 3-5cm on both sides).

Auscultation

Auscultate normal vesicular breath sounds, wheeze (COAD, asthma), crackles (bronchiectasis, pulmonary oedema), bronchial breath sounds (consolidation, cavity, broncho-pleural fistula), and vocal resonance.

Key points

◆ Look for signs of respiratory disease in general observation.
◆ Patients with COAD with right heart failure (cor pulmonale) may have peripheral oedema and a raised jugular venous pulse.

Station 3.9 Measuring equipment: temperature measurement

Information for the candidate

In this station your knowledge on equipment and the relevant physics of temperature measurement will be tested.

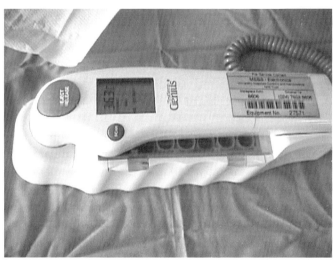

Figure 3.9.

Examiner's mark sheet

marks

Can you identify the equipment in Figure 3.9?   1 ☐

Tympanic membrane thermometer.

What is the principle behind its function?   2 ☐

It relies on the measurement of infrared radiation. The frequency of infrared light radiated from the tympanic membrane is measured.

What is its advantage?   1 ☐

It is quick and non-invasive.

Seek expert help if any patient with AF is known or found to have ventricular pre-excitation (WPW syndrome). Avoid using adenosine, diltiazem, verapamil, or digoxin in patients with pre-excited AF or atrial flutter as these drugs block the AV node and cause a relative increase in pre-excitation.

(For further reading please refer to the European resuscitation guidelines, 2005 - Peri-arrest arrhythmias).

Key points

♦ Atrial fibrillation in the ECG presents as irregular narrow complex tachycardia.
♦ Cardinal features suggesting decompensation are a reduced level of consciousness, hypotension (systolic pressure less than 90 mmHg), chest pain and heart failure.
♦ In stable patients, beta-blockers, digoxin and amiodarone are options.
♦ In unstable patients, synchronized DC shock is the treatment of choice.

Station 3.11 Anatomy: trigeminal nerve

Information for the candidate

In this station you will be asked about anatomy of a cranial nerve.

Examiner's mark sheet

marks

Which cranial nerve provides sensory innervation to the face?   1 ☐

Fifth cranial (trigeminal) nerve.

Describe the origin of the trigeminal nerve   1 ☐

It arises from the ventrolateral surface of the pons. It has a large sensory root and a small motor root.

What is the intracranial course of the roots soon after their origin?   1 ☐

About a centimetre after the origin the sensory root passes in a lateral and forward direction to enter Meckel's cave to form its ganglion.

What is the other name for this ganglion?   1 ☐

Semilunar or Gasserian ganglion.

Where is this ganglion located and what other structures is it related to?   4 ☐

It lies at the apex of the petrous temporal bone (Meckel's cave) and overlaps the foramen lacerum. The motor root of the trigeminal nerve and deep petrosal nerve pass deep to the ganglion. The temporal lobe is above the ganglion; the carotid artery lies medial to the ganglion. The cavernous sinus is posterior to the ganglion.

Name the three divisions of the trigeminal nerve   3 ☐

Ophthalmic, maxillary and mandibular.

State the course of the ophthalmic nerve   2 ☐

It passes through the superior orbital fissure, providing sensory innervation to the forehead and part of the lateral wall of the nose and septum (anterior and upper part).

- Inform the surgeon - request to stop any surgical stimuli.
- Call for senior help.
- If the vital signs are stable and no readily reversible cause is identified, send a blood gas for quick assessment of gas exchange, metabolic and electrolyte status.

The monitor shows a heart rate of 126/minute, a blood pressure of 190/120 mmHg, and a progressive ST segment depression. What would you do?

1×4 = 4

- Increase FIO_2.
- Ensure adequate plane of anaesthesia (end-tidal anaesthetic agent concentration; in total intravenous anaesthesia - check for pump, target concentration set and all connections).
- Ensure analgesia and wearing off from muscle relaxants.
- Control the ventilation to achieve normocarbia.

Despite the above measures ST segment depression and hypertension persists. Is there any other drug you would consider?

2

Glyceryl trinitrate (sublingual 0.3mg or an intravenous infusion 50mg/50ml of sodium chloride 0.9% - titrate to effect).

Even after optimizing fluid status, balanced anaesthesia and $EtCO_2$ the heart rate remains high at 140/minute. How would you manage tachycardia?

2

Beta blockade (esmolol: loading dose of 0.5mg/Kg followed by a maintenance dose of 50-150µg/Kg/minute. Alternatively, metoprolol or labetolol can be used).

How would you manage this patient postoperatively?   2 ☐

Further management depends on an obvious reversible cause of ischaemia, severity and duration, associated haemodynamic features and response to treatment. Ideally this patient should be looked after in the HDU. He will require a postoperative 12-lead ECG, surveillance for postoperative myocardial infarction and a cardiologist referral.

Total:	/20

Monitoring ECG

The ECG is a surface recording of the electrical activity of the myocardium. It is recorded by connecting various electrodes through which electrical potentials are measured. The ECG provides information on heart rate, rhythm and some indication of myocardial ischaemia.

The ECG monitoring system consists of the following three components:

- Skin electrodes detect the electrical activity of the heart.
- An amplifier to boost the ECG signal.
- An oscilloscope displays the amplified signal.

The ECG is recorded at a speed of 25mm per second and at a standardisation of 1cm height representing one mV of amplitude. On a standard ECG recording paper, width of a small square (1mm) represents 0.04 seconds and a large square (5mm) 0.2 seconds. Five big squares represent a time scale of 1 second and 300 big squares represent a time scale of 60 seconds or one minute. Hence if the rhythm is regular, heart rate can be calculated by dividing 300 by the number of big squares within one cardiac cycle (between two consecutive R waves).

The ECG lead system

There are 12 conventional leads, 6 in the frontal plane (I, II, III, aVR, aVL, aVF) and 6 in the horizontal plane (V1-V6). The heart is situated in the after the trauma. In chronic subdural haematomas, the clotted blood liquefies and appears as an isodense or hypodense (dark) area.

Key points

- Extradural haematomas commonly result from injury to the middle meningeal artery.
- On a CT scan, extradural haematomas have a characteristic biconvex shape.
- On a CT scan, acute subdural haematomas appear as a crescent-shaped hyperdense area.
- On a CT scan, chronic subdural haematomas may appear as an isodense or hypodense area.

Station 3.17 History taking: hernia repair

Information for the candidate

You are the anaesthetist allocated for a day-unit surgical list. You will be asked to take a 5-minute history as part of a pre-anaesthetic visit from a 60-year-old male patient. He is scheduled to have a hernia repair on your day-case list.

Examiner's mark sheet

marks

Introduces him/herself to the patient, confirms that he/she is talking to the right person and confirms the proposed surgery.	2 ☐
Previous anaesthetic history: appendicectomy.	1 ☐

Asks about cardiovascular disease

Chest pain: no.	1 ☐
Light-headedness/syncope/dizzy spells.	2 ☐
Shortness of breath on exertion.	1 ☐
Exercise tolerance (walks for half a mile, one flight of stairs).	2 ☐
Previous hospital admission for blackout.	1 ☐
Details of treatment for blackout (includes pacemaker).	2 ☐

Asks for the pacemaker card/details.	1	☐
Specifically asks for where and when recently tested.	2	☐
Hypertension.	1	☐
H/O smoking; 10 cigarettes a day.	1	☐
Smoker's cough.	1	☐
H/O alcohol intake: bottle of wine at weekends.	1	☐
H/O heartburn/reflux.	1	☐

Total:	/20

Information for the actor

You are 60 years old. You have been waiting for a hernia operation (lump in your left groin) for the past 2 years. You are scheduled to have the operation today. You will be interviewed by an anaesthetist. You are concerned that the hernia has started aching recently. You are hoping that it will be sorted out today.

Five years ago, following severe dizziness, you were admitted to hospital. As the heart was beating too slowly, a heart specialist inserted a pacemaker. Since then you never had any trouble with your heart, although you also have high blood pressure. You can walk for about half a mile before feeling short of breath. You live in a house and manage to climb upstairs at your own pace.

Your pacemaker was checked a year ago. You have smoked 10 cigarettes per day for the past 20 or more years. Consequently, you cough every morning and bring up some white phlegm.

When you were young you underwent an appendix operation with an uneventful general anaesthetic.

Key points

◆ Elicit the history of dizziness and ask for the details on investigations or treatment.
◆ Establish the reason for inserting the pacemaker.
◆ To ensure that the pacemaker is functioning normally, ask about regular follow-up checks.

(For more information please refer to OSCE set 1, station 1.12).

Station 3.18 Anaesthetic equipment: entonox valve

Information for the candidate

This is a station on physics and equipment used in anaesthetic practice.

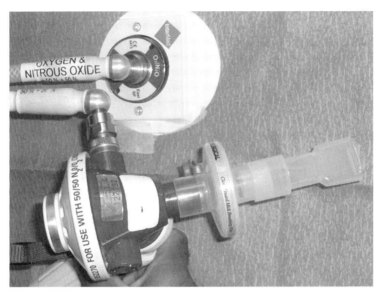

Figure 3.18.

Examiner's mark sheet

	marks
Identify this equipment	1 ☐
Entonox valve.	
What is the pressure in the entonox cylinder?	1 ☐
137 bar (13700 kPa).	

State how entonox is formed   2 ☐

Oxygen gas is bubbled through liquid nitrous oxide; during the process nitrous oxide vaporises and a gaseous mixture is formed.

What is the critical temperature of the gas mixture in this cylinder?   1 ☐

The critical temperature of the mixture is decreased to -7°C (pseudocritical temperature); below this temperature liquefaction and separation of the two components occur.

What is the Poynting effect?   1 ☐

The effect describes the process of dissolving oxygen in nitrous oxide liquid. The gaseous oxygen is bubbled through the liquid nitrous oxide. Liquid nitrous oxide vaporises to form a gaseous oxygen-nitrous oxide mixture. This is called the Poynting effect. The critical temperature and pressure of a gas may be affected when it is mixed with another gas. In a cylinder of entonox, the new critical temperature of the mixture (known as the pseudocritical temperature) changes to approximately -5.5 to -7°C.

What would the problem be of storing the cylinder at a very low temperature, e.g. -10°C?   2 ☐

The gases separate; initially a high concentration of oxygen is delivered and later a high concentration of nitrous oxide is delivered.

At what temperature would these gases separate in a pipe line at 4 bar?   1 ☐

Even lower; -30°C.

What precautions should be taken during storage of this cylinder?   2 ☐

It should be stored horizontally, at a temperature above 5°C for 24 hours before use. (The purpose of the horizontal position is to enhance the area for diffusion. Alternatively, the cylinder can be used before 24 hours by repeated inversion).

How does this pressure relief valve differ from others?   2 ☐

It is a two-stage pressure demand regulator valve. The first one is a pressure-reducing valve and the second one is a demand valve which allows gas to flow when the pressure is reduced below atmospheric level.

Name some clinical uses of entonox   2 ☐

Labour analgesia, pain relief in casualty (ureteric colic, sickle crisis, prehospital analgesia), wound dressing in burns.

What advice would you give for its use during labour?   2 ☐

It takes about 30 seconds to act and the analgesic effect lasts for 60 seconds after discontinuing. The mother should inhale when the contraction begins, to ensure the peak effect at the height of the contraction.

What are the contra-indications for its use?   2 ☐

Bowel obstruction, pneumothorax, intracranial air (early postoperative period following craniotomy), and vitamin B12 deficiency (as prolonged use can cause bone marrow suppression).

What is the maximum recommended concentration of nitrous oxide in the theatre atmosphere?   1 ☐

25 ppm.

| Total: | /20 |

Entonox

Entonox is 50% oxygen and 50% nitrous oxide by volume. The mixture is prepared by bubbling oxygen through liquid nitrous oxide. The cylinders are coloured blue with blue-white quartered shoulders. They are supplied at a pressure of 137 bar.

The critical temperature is the temperature above which a gas cannot be liquefied, however much pressure is applied. The critical pressure is the minimum pressure that causes liquefaction at a critical temperature. The critical temperature of oxygen is -18°C and of nitrous oxide is 36.5°C. The pseudocritical temperature is the temperature at which the gas mixture separates into their component parts. For an entonox cylinder (at 137 bar) this is -7°C; for an entonox pipeline (at 4 bar) it is -30°C. Hence, the cylinders must be stored above the pseudocritical temperature (-7°C) to prevent liquefaction of nitrous oxide. As the gases separate, initially an oxygen-rich mixture will be delivered followed by nitrous oxide rich gas. Warming and thorough mixing of the constituents can avoid this problem.

Entonox is useful in labour analgesia, during a change of dressings for burns and other minor procedures. As nitrous oxide can quickly occupy and enlarge air-containing cavities, it should be avoided in the presence of a pneumothorax, bowel obstruction, etc. Prolonged use of entonox is not encouraged in view of the effect of nitrous oxide on the methionine synthase system and on bone marrow.

Key points

♦ Entonox is a compressed gas mixture containing 50% oxygen and 50% nitrous oxide by volume.

♦ The valve for entonox is a special two-staged pressure demand regulator.

♦ Below the pseudocritical temperature, liquefaction of nitrous oxide and separation of the two components can occur.

♦ Fast onset and short duration of action has made it popular for short-term pain relief. It is not recommended for prolonged use.

Station 3.19 Technical skill: intra-osseous infusion

Information for the candidate

In this station your technical skill on using an intra-osseous needle will be tested.

Examiner's mark sheet

marks

What is the indication for intra-osseous infusion of fluids?   2   ☐

In children under the age of approximately 6 years, when venous access is difficult (more than 3 attempts), the intra-osseous route is an option for resuscitation.

Can you demonstrate how you would perform intra-osseous puncture?   1 x 8   ☐
=8

♦ Checks appropriate needle (intra-osseous needle or bone marrow aspiration needle).

♦ Position: sufficient padding under the knee and about 30° flexion of the knee.

- Puncture site: anteromedial surface of the proximal tibia; one fingerbreadth below the tibial tubercle.
- Local anaesthetic to the puncture site.
- Needle insertion: initially inserts the needle at 90° to skin; after approaching the bone redirects the needle 45° to 00° caudally.
- Uses a twisting motion to enter the bone marrow.
- Removes the stylet and attaches the needle to a 10ml syringe.
- Aspirates bone marrow and injects saline.

Why should the needle be directed caudally?   1 [   ]

This direction is to avoid the epiphyseal growth plate.

How would you confirm the correct placement of the   3 [   ]
needle?

- Aspiration of bone marrow.
- Needle is firm and remains upright.
- On injecting saline, there is no resistance and no evidence of swelling.

What are the complications?   4 [   ]

- Subcutaneous and subperiosteal infusion.
- Epiphyseal plate injury.
- Haematoma.
- Infection.
- Pressure necrosis of the skin.

State two relative contra-indications for intra-osseous 2 [   ]
infusion

- Fracture of the involved bone.
- Osteomyclitis.

Total:	/20

Intra-osseous infusion

Intra-osseous infusion is one of the quickest ways to establish access for the rapid infusion of fluids, drugs and blood products in emergency situations as well as for resuscitation. It is popular in paediatric resuscitation. The marrow cavity is in continuity with the venous circulation and can therefore be used to infuse fluids and drugs, and to take blood samples for cross-match. Placement of an intra-osseous needle is indicated when vascular access is needed in life-threatening situations in infants and children under the age of 6 years. It is indicated when attempts at venous access fail (3 futile attempts or more than 90 seconds). Although principally advocated for use in young children, it has been successfully used in older children where the iliac crest may also be used. It is advised not to use the technique in a fractured bone and in the presence of osteomyelitis.

An intra-osseous infusion needle or bone marrow needle is used to access the space. Although there are different needle sizes, 14 and 16G are generally used. The best site to use is the flat anteromedial aspect of the tibia. The anterior aspect of the femur and the superior iliac crest can also be used. The tibia is preferred since the anteromedial aspect of the bone lies just under the skin and is easily identified.

To perform the technique, palpate the tibial tuberosity. The site for cannulation lies 1-3cm below this tuberosity on the anteromedial surface of the tibia. Take all aseptic precautions. If the child is awake, inject local anaesthetic in the skin and infiltrate down to the periosteum. Flex the knee and have a support behind the knee. Insert the intra-osseous needle at 90° to the skin (perpendicular) and slightly caudal to avoid the epiphysial growth plate. Advance the needle using a drilling motion. Feeling a 'give' implies penetration of the cortex of the bone. Remove the trochar and confirm the position by aspirating blood. Inject saline 0.9% to ensure there is no resistance and there is no local swelling. The needle is secured in place with a sterile dressing.

Notable complications are tibial fracture, haematoma, osteomyelitis and skin necrosis. The longer the needle is left in place, the higher the risks will be. But, in general, it is a safe and life-saving technique. Fluids can be infused manually by injecting through a 50ml syringe or through a pressurised infusion bag.

Key points

- Intra-osseous infusion is a life-saving temporary emergency measure.
- It is indicated in emergency situations when intravenous access fails.
- Use an aseptic technique.
- The anteromedial aspect of the upper tibia is often used.
- The port can be used to aspirate blood for investigations and to infuse fluids for resuscitation.
- Complication rates are low if aseptic precautions are taken, but remove it as soon as possible once definitive venous access is secured.

Station 3.20 Technical skill: intravenous regional anaesthesia

Information for the candidate

A 60-year-old female patient is scheduled for manipulation of a Colles' fracture of the left wrist. You will be asked to describe the steps in performing Bier's block (intravenous regional anaesthesia).

Examiner's mark sheet

marks

Rules out contra-indications for Bier's block (allergy to drugs   2   ☐
local anaesthetics, sickle cell disease).

Ensures that resuscitation facilities are available (airway   2   ☐
equipment, drugs).

Monitors ECG, SpO_2, NIBP.   2   ☐

Inserts the intravenous cannula in the opposite arm. 2 ☐

Inserts the cannula in the same arm. 2 ☐

Measures baseline blood pressure. 2 ☐

Exsanguinates the arm. 2 ☐

Inflates the tourniquet to a pressure 100mmHg above systolic 2 ☐
blood pressure.

Injects the calculated amount of local anaesthetic (prilocaine 2 ☐
or lidocaine).

Deflates the tourniquet only after 20 minutes at least. 2 ☐

Total: /20

Intravenous regional anaesthesia (IVRA)

IVRA is indicated for any procedure on the upper limb below the elbow or lower limb below the knee that can be completed within 45-60 minutes. With this technique the onset of anaesthesia is rapid. The technique is best avoided if a tourniquet cannot be used safely, as in vascular insufficiency and sickle cell disease. As with all other local anaesthetic blocks, resuscitation equipment should be immediately available.

The recommended drug for IVRA is prilocaine, as among the local anaesthetics it has minimal toxicity and a high therapeutic index. Lidocaine is an acceptable alternative. Adrenaline should not be added. Bupivacaine is not suitable in view of cardiotoxicity. A suitable dose to use in an arm is about 40ml of 0.5% prilocaine or 0.5% lidocaine. The maximum recommended dose for prilocaine is 3-6mg/Kg and it is 3mg/Kg for lidocaine.

Prior to performing the block, the patient's baseline blood pressure is measured. Intravenous cannulae are secured, one for the block and another one for vascular access in case of any complication. Vital signs are monitored. The tourniquet is then applied to the upper arm or thigh over a layer of cotton roll. Exsanguination of blood from the limb prior to inflation of the tourniquet aids in a better block. This is done with an Esmarch rubber bandage or by simple elevation of the limb with the corresponding artery compressed. The tourniquet is then inflated to a pressure of 50-100 mm Hg above the systolic blood pressure.

After about 5-10 minutes, patients may start experiencing tourniquet pain due to pressure from the tourniquet. This may be avoided by using a double tourniquet technique. In this method two tourniquets are placed on the patient's arm or thigh. Initially, the more proximal (upper) tourniquet is inflated and the local anaesthetic is injected. After about 5 minutes, the distal (lower) tourniquet is inflated (over the numb area) and then the proximal one is deflated.

When used with routine precautions, IVRA is a safe technique with few complications. The most important complication is the risk of local anaesthetic toxicity in the event of inadvertent deflation of the tourniquet soon after the local anaesthetic has been injected. These will range from light-headedness and tinnitus to muscle twitching, loss of consciousness and convulsions. Serious cardiac side effects are rare.

Key points

♦ Ensure the patient is fasted and other routine pre-anaesthetic assessments are performed.
♦ Ensure a minimum standard monitoring.
♦ Resuscitation drugs and equipment should be prepared.
♦ The double-tourniquet technique helps to minimise tourniquet pain.
♦ Prilocaine 0.5% or lidocaine 0.5% are commonly used.
♦ It is a safe technique provided the correct dose of local anaesthetic is used, tourniquet pressure is carefully monitored and resuscitation equipment is immediately available.

OSCE
set 4

Station 4.1 Anaesthetic equipment: Bain breathing system

Information for the candidate

You are performing an anaesthetic machine check, as you do routinely at the beginning of a list. In this station you will be asked to assemble all the components of a breathing system and to check the system to ensure that it is safe to use.

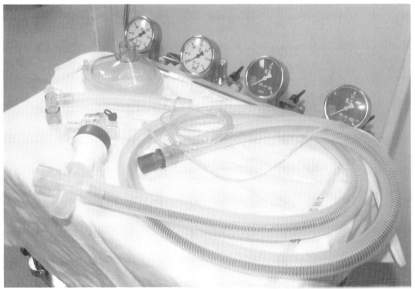

Figure 4.1a Components of a breathing system.

Examiner's mark sheet

marks

Connects all the components correctly. 3 ☐

Connects the proximal end to the common gas outlet. 1 ☐

Visually inspects the outer tubing. 1 ☐

Sets the fresh gas flow (FGF) on the anaesthetic machine at 5L/minute. 1 ☐

Confirms the flow into the system by occluding the tube at the patient end and ensures that the reservoir bag fills, turns off the flow meter and ensures that the reservoir bag does not collapse. 2 ☐

Makes sure that the inner tube is not disconnected, sets the gas flow at 5L/min, then occludes the inner tube using a plunger of a 2ml syringe, and the bobbin should dip due to back pressure. 2 ☐

Checks the function of the APL valve. 2 ☐

Checks the filter and angle piece for any defect or blockage. 2 ☐

What happens if the inner tube is disconnected at the machine end? 2 ☐

This increases the dead space resulting in hypercapnia and hypoxaemia.

What is the FGF required for spontaneous ventilation for avoiding re-breathing? 2 ☐

A fresh gas flow of 150-250ml/Kg or 2-3 times a minute ventilation is required during spontaneous ventilation to prevent re-breathing.

What should be the FGF during controlled ventilation to maintain normocapnia?

2 ☐

During controlled ventilation, a flow of 70-100ml/Kg/minute is required to maintain normocapnia.

Total:	/20

Information for the examiner

The anaesthetic machine has already been checked. The Bain breathing system needs to be correctly assembled. The candidate is expected to connect the gas sampling line correctly in the breathing filter.

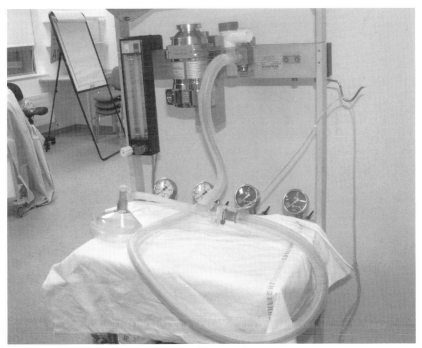

Figure 4.1b Assembled Bain breathing system.

Bain breathing system

The Bain breathing system is a coaxial version of the Mapleson D system. The components of the Bain breathing system include an inner tube, outer tube, APL valve and a reservoir bag. The inner tube (7mm internal diameter) carries fresh gas flow and the outer tube (22mm internal diameter) carries expired gas. Disconnection of the inner tube at the machine end leads to increased dead space and kinking of the inner tube results in obstruction to the flow of fresh gas. The amount of rebreathing depends on the fresh gas flow. Fresh gas flow must be high enough to purge the exhaled gas from the outer tubing and to supplement the stored fresh gas in the outer tube so that during the next inspiration, mixed gas from the reservoir bag does not reach the patient.

The breathing system should be checked for integrity and any obstruction of both the inner and outer tubes. In order to check the integrity of the inner tube, the lumen of the inner tubing should be occluded with a finger or the plunger of a 2ml syringe. A rise in gas pressure within the anaesthetic circuit leads to downward movement of the bobbin in the flow meter. Another test that can be used for ensuring the integrity of the inner tube is the Pethick test. The APL valve should be closed, the reservoir bag and breathing system should be filled using an oxygen flush, and the patient end of the breathing system should be occluded. While activating the oxygen flush, the occlusion at the patient end should be released. Due to the Venturi effect at the patient end, fresh gas flow from the outer tubing and reservoir bag is entrained. Therefore, the reservoir bag collapses.

The Bain breathing system is less efficient for spontaneous ventilation as it requires high fresh gas flow. During controlled ventilation, a longer expiratory phase and expiratory pause, allows the outer tube to be filled with fresh gas flow. A fresh gas flow of 70-80ml/Kg/minute (6-7L/minute) will maintain a normal arterial CO_2 tension (normocapnia) and a flow of 100ml/Kg/minute is required for mild hypocapnia.

The Bain breathing system has low dead space and offers low resistance to breathing. Fresh gas in the inner tube is warmed up to some extent as it passes through the expiratory limb (outer tube).

Key points

- The Bain breathing system is a coaxial version of the Mapleson D system.
- Disconnection of the inner tube leads to increased dead space and hypercapnia.
- It is an efficient system for controlled ventilation.

Station 4.2 Data interpretation: lung function tests

Information for the candidate

In this station you will be assessed on your knowledge and understanding of interpretation of lung function tests.

A 70-year-old female patient is scheduled to have a total knee replacement. She smokes 10-20 cigarettes per day and gives a history of shortness of breath on exertion. As part of her pre-operative assessment, the following lung function tests are performed.

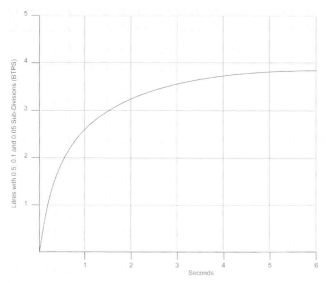

Figure 4.2a Lung function test.

Vitalograph

The vitalograph is a type of dry spirometer, and is portable and suitable for bedside use. FEV1 is the volume recorded at the end of the first second during forced expiration and the FVC is the total volume recorded at the end of forced expiration following a deep inspiration.

The vitalograph is useful in distinguishing obstructive lung disease from restrictive lung disease. In restrictive lung disease, both FEV1 and FVC are reduced; therefore the ratio of FEV1: FVC remains normal or high. In obstructive lung disease, FEV1 is reduced in comparison to FVC resulting in a low FEV1: FVC ratio.

The peak expiratory flow rate (PEFR) can be calculated from the initial gradient of the trace. PEFR is usually normal in restrictive lung disease. PEFR is reduced in obstructive lung disease, such as asthma and chronic obstructive airway disease.

The flow volume loop helps to distinguish obstructive lung disease from restrictive lung disease in addition to distinguishing intrathoracic airway obstruction from extrathoracic airway obstruction.

In fixed obstruction of a large airway, the maximum airflow is limited both in inspiration and expiration; both phases are flattened (Figure 4.2c).

In variable intrathoracic airway obstruction, as in asthma, narrowing of the airway is maximal in expiration. The flow-volume loop shows a greater reduction of flow in the expiratory phase (Figure 4.2d).

In variable extrathoracic airway obstruction, narrowing of the airway is maximal during inspiration. The flow volume loop shows a greater reduction of flow in the inspiratory phase.

The density of helium is lower than that of nitrogen or oxygen; it reduces the Reynolds number and therefore should alter the flow from turbulent to laminar in the larger airways. It effectively overcomes the airway resistance and improves the flow in upper airway obstruction. Recent research supports its use in COAD and asthma.

Heliox is supplied as a mixture of 21% oxygen and 79% helium in a black cylinder with white and brown quarters on the shoulder of the cylinder.

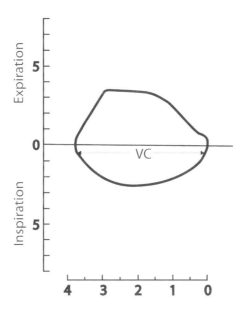

Figure 4.2c Fixed large airway obstruction.

Block of the left anterior hemi-fascicle is characterised by left axis deviation in the absence of inferior myocardial infarction or other cause of left axis deviation. Block of the left posterior hemi-fascicle is characterised by right axis deviation. Bifascicular block is the combination of right bundle branch block and left anterior or posterior hemiblock. Bifascicular block in association with first degree heart block is known as trifascicular block.

ECG criteria for left ventricular hypertrophy

- Depth of the S wave in V1 and height of the R wave in V5 or V6 should be more than 35mm.
- R wave in V4, V5 or V6 more than 30mm.
- S wave in V1, V2, V3 more than 30mm.
- R wave in aVL more than 13mm.

Indications for implantation of a permanent pacemaker

The following are indications where there is evidence and/or general agreement that pacing is beneficial:

- Third degree AV block associated with bradycardia, documented asystole of more than 3 seconds or an escape rate <40bpm.
- Second degree AV block associated with symptomatic bradycardia.
- Sinus node dysfunction with documented symptomatic bradycardia.
- Symptomatic bifascicular or trifascicular heart block.
- Persistent second degree AV block or third degree AV block following acute myocardial infarction.

Blood supply

The right coronary artery provides blood supply to the SA node in 60% of patients and the AV node in 80% of patients. The left bundle branch usually receives blood from the left anterior descending branch of the left coronary artery. The right bundle branch receives most of its blood from septal perforators of the left anterior descending artery. There may also be a collateral blood supply from the right coronary artery or left circumflex artery.

Key points

- A prolonged PR interval of more than 0.2 seconds indicates first degree heart block.
- A widened QRS complex with a rSR pattern in leads V1 and V2 is seen in right bundle branch block.
- The left bundle branch receives blood supply from the left anterior descending artery.
- Left bundle branch block indicates organic heart disease.
- Right bundle branch block with left anterior hemiblock is the commonest form of bifascicular block.

Station 4.4 Data interpretation: vital parameters

Information for the candidate

A 64-year-old female underwent an elective left hemicolectomy 3 days ago. Her blood pressure is low and peripheral oxygen saturation is 91% while on 40% oxygen supplementation. Patient controlled analgesia (PCA) with morphine has been prescribed postoperatively. On clinical examination, the respiratory rate is 22 per minute, heart rate is 120/minute, and blood pressure is 90/40 mmHg. You are now presented with a set of charts and blood results on the ward.

- Urea: 12.4mmol/L, creatinine: 118µmol/L, Na^+: 142mmol/L, K^+: 4.8mmol/L.

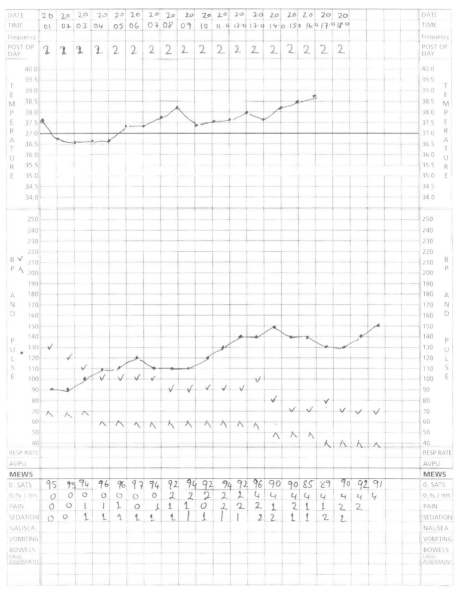

Pain score

0	No pain
1	Mild pain
2	Moderate pain
3	Severe pain

Sedation score

Awake and alert
Occasionally drowsy
Frequently drowsy but easily rousable
Unrousable

Figure 4.4a Observation chart.

24 HOUR FLUID BALANCE CHART

Name
Hospital No

Ward

Instructions for next 24 hours

Previous days fluid balance =

INTAKE

TIME	ORAL VOLUME	ORAL TOTAL	INTRAVENOUS FLUID	IV VOLUME	IV TOTAL	NG/NJ/PEG FLUID	NG VOLUME	NG TOTAL	OTHER
01:00			5% Dextrose	500					
02:00				100					
03:00				120					
04:00				80					
05:00				100					
06:00				100	1000				
07:00			Nacl 0.9%	80					
08:00				80					
09:00				60					
10:00				60					
11:00				60					
12:00				60					
13:00				80	1480				
14:00				80					
15:00				60					
16:00				80					
17:00				80					
18:00									
19:00									
20:00									
21:00									
22:00									
23:00									
24:00									
TOTAL =			TOTAL =			TOTAL =			

OUTPUT

TIME	URINE VOLUME	URINE TOTAL	ASPIRATE OR VOMIT VOLUME	TOTAL	STOMA/BOWELS VOLUME	TOTAL	OTHER VOLUME	TOTAL
01:00	70		0					
02:00	80		0					
03:00	90		80					
04:00	30		120					
05:00	40		80					
06:00	20	330	130	410				
07:00	20		50					
08:00	10		80					
09:00	30		100					
10:00	20		120					
11:00	15		80					
12:00	0	425	110	950				
13:00	0		0					
14:00	10		90					
15:00	15		110					
16:00	20		100					
17:00	15	485	80	1330				
18:00								
19:00								
20:00								
21:00								
22:00								
23:00								
24:00								
TOTAL =			TOTAL =		TOTAL =		TOTAL =	

TOTAL INTAKE = _____
TOTAL OUTPUT = _____
FLUID BALANCE = _____

Figure 4.4b 24-hour fluid balance chart.

Examiner's mark sheet

Please tick the correct answer - true or false   **marks**

1. The most likely cause of low oxygen saturation is True False 2 ☐
   opioid-induced respiratory depression.
2. This patient is likely to be hypovolaemic.   True False 2 ☐
3. This patient has had adequate pain relief during the True False 2 ☐
   last six hours.
4. Renal parameters suggest pre-renal renal failure.   True False 2 ☐
5. Intravenous furosemide should be given True False 2 ☐
   immediately.
6. Arterial blood gas will reveal respiratory acidosis. True False 2 ☐
7. At 13:00 hours the measured fluid loss is 1915ml.   True False 2 ☐
8. Urine osmolality is likely to be less than True False 2 ☐
   320mOsm/Kg.
9. Inspired oxygen concentration should be increased   True False 2 ☐
   to 100% immediately.
10. This patient is likely to need a laparotomy.   True False 2 ☐

Total: /20

Answers

1. False. The pain score indicates that the patient is in pain. The PCA
   chart (not available) would indicate total dose of morphine received.

2. True. Total intravenous fluid intake over 17 hours is 1780ml and the
   measured output is 1815ml. The patient is pyrexial, there will be
   further insensible loss and therefore this patient is in negative fluid
   balance.

3. False. The pain score varies between 1 to 2 (mild to moderate).

4. True. A raised serum urea level and hypovolaemia suggests pre-renal
   renal failure.

5. False. Intravascular fluid volume and renal perfusion should be optimised.

6. False. An arterial blood gas will reveal respiratory alkalosis.

7. False. At 13:00 hours the measured fluid loss is 1375ml.

8. False. In pre-renal type renal failure osmolality is normal (more than 450mOsm/Kg). Urine osmolality is likely to be less than 310mOsm/Kg in renal tubular acidosis.

9. True. Inspired oxygen concentration should be increased to 100% immediately.

10. True.

This patient underwent major abdominal surgery and is hypotensive, hypoxic and oliguric during the postoperative period. Causes of hypotension in this patient could be hypovolaemia, peripheral vasodilation from a systemic inflammatory response or sepsis, and a reduced cardiac output due to myocardial depression.

The observation chart indicates that the patient has mild to moderate pain. Her respiratory rate is high. Therefore, the patient is more likely to have respiratory alkalosis rather than respiratory acidosis. Hypotension and a reduced tissue perfusion can result in metabolic acidosis.

Key points

◆ Careful evaluation of the observation chart and fluid balance chart is essential prior to making decisions.
◆ The majority of surgical patients are likely to be hypovolaemic during the early postoperative period.
◆ Patients with sepsis require optimum fluid therapy and vasopressor/ inotropic support to improve organ function.

Station 4.5 Anatomy: the orbit and ophthalmic anaesthesia

Information for the candidate

In this station you will be asked questions on the anatomy of the orbit and the technical skill of performing eye blocks will be assessed.

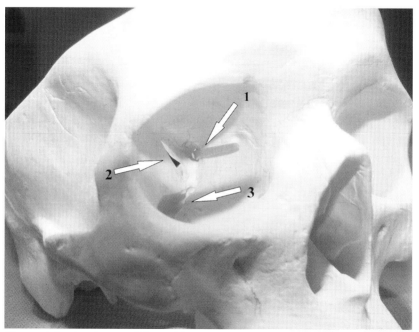

Figure 4.5a Anatomy of the orbit.

Examiner's mark sheet

marks

Name the foramen labelled 1 in Figure 4.5a   1

Optic foramen.

What structures pass through this foramen? 1 ☐

Optic nerve and ophthalmic artery.

Name the structure labelled 2 in Figure 4.5a 1 ☐

Superior orbital fissure.

What structures pass through this fissure? 3 ☐

Lacrimal. frontal, nasociliary, oculomotor, trochlear and abducens nerves, and the superior ophthalmic vein.

Name the structure labelled 3 in Figure 4.5a 1 ☐

Inferior orbital fissure.

What is the normal axial length of the eye ball and what is the significance? 2 ☐

Normal axial length is 22-26mm. An axial length of more than 26mm suggests a large eye and hence there is a risk of globe puncture during peribulbar and retrobulbar block.

Describe the motor nerve supply to the extra-ocular muscles 2 ☐

- Lateral rectus is supplied by the abducens nerve.
- Superior oblique is supplied by the trochlear nerve.
- Other extraocular muscles: medial rectus, inferior rectus, superior rectus and inferior oblique are all supplied by the oculomotor nerve.

The axial length of the eyeball is measured from the external corneal surface to the retina. An axial length of more than 26mm denotes a large eye and increases the risk of globe perforation during peribulbar block.

The motor nerve supply to the extra-ocular muscles is by the 3rd, 4th and 6th cranial nerves. The superior oblique is supplied by the 4th cranial nerve and the lateral rectus is supplied by the 6th cranial nerve. The remainder of the muscles are supplied by the 3rd cranial nerve. A mnemonic is LR6 SO4.

Eye blocks

In retrobulbar block, the needle is inserted into the intraconal space behind the globe. As the local anaesthetic is deposited close to the motor and sensory nerves, a small volume (1.5-4ml) of local anaesthetic is adequate to produce a satisfactory block.

In peribulbar block, the needle is placed outside the muscle cone, further away from the apex. A larger volume of local anaesthetic (6-10ml) is required to produce satisfactory block.

In sub-Tenon's block, Tenon's capsule is elevated from the sclera and local anaesthetic is deposited into the sub-Tenon's (episcleral) space.

Local anaesthetic drugs

Lidocaine hydrochloride 2% and bupivacaine hydrochloride 0.5-0.75% are the commonly used local anaesthetics. Duration of lidocaine can be prolonged by the addition of epinephrine. Longer duration of bupivacaine provides postoperative pain relief.

Benoxinate 0.4% solution and amethocaine 0.5% solution are used for topical anaesthesia.

Epinephrine causes vasoconstriction, delays the absorption of local anaesthetic and prolongs the duration of action. The preferred concentration is 1:200,000 (5μg/ml). The total dose should not exceed 0.2mg.

Hyaluronidase breaks down the collagen bonds and facilitates diffusion of local anaesthetic across the connective tissue septal barriers. It is used in a concentration of 7.5 to 15 units/ml.

Complications of sub-Tenon's block include pain on injection, subconjuctival haemorrhage, chemosis and the potential for damaging one of the vortex veins. Peripheral orbit anaesthesia may be incomplete with sub-Tenon's block.

Complications related to ophthalmic regional block

- Retrobulbar haemorrhage.
- Subconjuctival haemorrhage.
- Subconjuctival oedema (chemosis).
- Optic nerve damage.
- Globe perforation.
- Intravascular injection.
- Central spread of local anaesthetic: clinical features include drowsiness, vomiting, convulsions, cardiorespiratory arrest.
- Oculocardiac reflex due to traction on the eye, rapid distension of tissues by local anaesthetic or by haemorrhage.

Key points

- The optic nerve, ophthalmic artery and central retinal vein pass through the optic foramen.
- Lacrimal, frontal and trochlear (LFT) nerves pass through the superior orbital fissure and lie outside the muscle cone.
- The inferior orbital fissure transmits the infra-orbital (maxillary) nerve, infra-orbital artery and infra-orbital vein.

Station 4.8 Clinical examination: airway examination

Information for the candidate

A 75-year-old male patient has presented for an inguinal hernia repair as a day-case surgical procedure. As part of the pre-operative assessment you have been asked to perform a clinical examination of the airway.

Examiner's mark sheet

marks

Introduces him/herself to the patient and explains his/her role.   1 ☐

Inspects the front and side of the neck.   2 ☐

Elicits mouth opening and measures inter-incisor distance.   2 ☐

Asks the patient to protrude their mandible (forward movement of the lower jaw).   1 ☐

Performs the Mallampati test.   1 ☐

Correctly measures the sternomental distance.   1 ☐

Correctly measures the thyromental distance.   1 ☐

Assesses the full range of neck movements.   2 ☐

Checks for patency of nasal passages.   1 ☐

What would you see and what information would you obtain from a Mallampati test?   4 ☐

Depending on the pharyngeal structures visualised, four classes are described:

◈ Class 1: faucial pillars, soft palate and uvula seen.
◈ Class 2: faucial pillars and soft palate seen. The base of the tongue masks the uvula.

- ◆ Class 3: only the soft palate is visible.
- ◆ Class 4: even the soft palate is not visible; only the hard palate is seen.

Class 3 and 4 are caused by difficulty in extending the head, opening the mouth or by a large tongue. A higher score indicates a possible difficult laryngoscopy.

What are the risk factors included in Wilson risk sum scoring?

3

It includes 5 predictive factors, each scored on a three-point scale (0-2): weight, head and neck movement, jaw movement, receding mandible and buck teeth.

What is the significance of this scoring system?

1

A total score of 2 or more is associated with an increased incidence of difficult intubation.

Total:	/20

Airway assessment

Airway assessment includes history, examination and investigation. This is a clinical examination station and you are asked to assess the airway as part of the pre-anaesthetic assessment.

On inspection any gross abnormality of the face, mouth, head and neck should be obvious. Inspect both from the front and sides of the patient. Any scars from previous surgery and swelling around the head neck region should be noted.

On fully opening the mouth, the distance between the incisors varies from 4-6cm. A rough estimate is the patient's own two or three fingers aligned vertically to accommodate the gap.

What are the adverse effects of amiodarone? 2 ☐

It causes hypotension and bradycardia.

What is the differential diagnosis? 2 ☐

Supraventricular tachycardia with bundle branch block.

How would you treat previously confirmed supra- 2 ☐
ventricular tachycardia (SVT) with bundle branch block?

Adenosine 6mg intravenous rapid bolus; if unsuccessful,
12mg bolus; if still unsuccessful, administer a further 12mg.

If this patient is unstable what treatment would you 2 ☐
instigate?

Unstable SVT is treated with synchronised cardioversion,
starting with 200J monophasic or 120-150J biphasic energy.
If this fails, increase the energy in increments (360J for
monophasic, 200J or higher with biphasic).

| Total: | /20 |

Management of broad complex tachycardia

In broad complex tachycardia, the QRS complexes are more than 0.12
seconds in duration. Regular broad complex tachycardia is most likely
ventricular tachycardia or SVT with bundle branch block. In a stable
patient it should be treated with amiodarone and in an unstable patient it
should be treated with synchronised cardioversion.

Irregular broad complex tachycardia is more likely AF with bundle branch
block. Another possible cause is AF with ventricular pre-excitation (Wolff-
Parkinson-White syndrome).

Amiodarone is used to treat stable ventricular tachycardia (VT), polymorphic VT, broad complex tachycardia of uncertain origin, paroxysmal SVT uncontrolled by other measures and to control ventricular rate in pre-excited atrial arrhythmias. The loading dose of amiodarone is 300mg given over 20-60 minutes, and can be followed by infusion of 900mg over 24 hours. An additional dose of 150mg can be repeated as required to a maximum daily dose of 2g. Major adverse effects are hypotension and bradycardia which can be prevented by reducing the rate of infusion. Amiodarone causes thrombophlebitis when administered through peripheral veins. Whenever possible it should be given through a central venous catheter.

In ventricular pre-excitation, drugs that block AV conduction should be avoided. These include adenosine, digoxin, verapamil and diltiazem.

Key points

- Broad complex tachycardia in an unstable patient should be treated with synchronised cardioversion.
- Broad complex tachycardia in a stable patient can be treated with amiodarone.
- The maximum dose of amiodarone is 2g in 24 hours.

Station 4.11 Anatomy: larynx

Information for the candidate

In this station you will be asked questions on the anatomy of the larynx.

oropharynx and posterior two thirds of the tongue need to be anaesthetised before performing this block.

With translaryngeal anaesthesia, the skin over the cricothyroid membrane is infiltrated with local anaesthetic. Then a needle or cannula attached to a syringe containing normal saline is inserted through the cricothyroid membrane; the needle should be directed backwards and caudad to avoid trauma to the vocal cords. Correct placement is confirmed by aspiration of air via the needle. 2-4ml of 4% lidocaine should be injected at the end of inspiration. During the process the patient coughs and anaesthesia should spread both above and below the cords. Complications such as a haematoma, a broken needle and infection have been reported as a result of nerve block, but they are rare.

Key points

- In infants, the glottis is situated opposite the 3rd and 4th cervical inter-vertebral space.
- In children it is located opposite the 4th and 5th cervical inter-vertebral space.
- In adults, the glottis is situated at the level of the 5th cervical vertebra.
- In adults, the cricoid cartilage is located at the level of the 6th cervical vertebra.
- If the recurrent laryngeal nerve is partially damaged, adductors override the abductor and the vocal cord becomes fixed in the midline.
- Bilateral damage of the recurrent laryngeal nerve may result in complete airway obstruction.

Station 4.12 History taking: tympanoplasty

Information for the candidate

In this station you will be asked to take a history from a patient who is scheduled to have a tympanoplasty.

Examiner's mark sheet

marks

Introduces him/herself, explains his/her role and confirms that he/she is talking to the right person.   1 ☐

Confirms the nature and reason for the proposed surgery (hearing loss).   1 ☐

Previous anaesthetic history.   1 ☐

Details about previous operation.   1 ☐

Elicits past H/O sarcoidosis.   1 ☐

Enquires about progression of sarcoidosis and presence of cough.   1 ☐

Exercise tolerance.   2 ☐

Asks about lung function tests.   1 ☐

Past medical H/O CVA.   1 ☐

Further details on CVA (investigations, full recovery).   2 ☐

H/O hypertension.   1 ☐

Drug history: steroids: prednisolone, stopped a year ago.   2 ☐

Aspirin 75mg per day; antihypertensive: perindopril 4mg once a day.   2 ☐

Social history: smoking/alcohol.   1 ☐

Asks about dentures, crowns and caps.   1 ☐

A structured approach of gathering information.   1 ☐

Total:	/20

Information for the actor

You are 65 years old. You have been having a problem with your left ear for some time. You had an ear infection 2 years ago which left you with a hole in the ear drum of your left ear. You have been waiting to have an operation on the left ear.

You also have a few other health-related problems; they are not your concern now, so do not volunteer further information unless the doctor asks you specific questions. You had a mild stroke 5 years ago; however, you have recovered completely. You have been suffering from sarcoidosis (a condition that produces tiny lumps of cells in various organs of the body, mainly involving the lungs; diagnosed 10 years ago). Your lungs have been mildly affected and you feel perfectly alright now. In the past you were taking steroid tablets (prednisolone) for the sarcoidosis, but your doctor asked you to stop these tablets a year ago. You do not have a cough any more and you feel fit and healthy, except for the trouble with your hearing.

You also suffer from high blood pressure; you have a regular blood pressure check with your doctor and it is under control. You take tablets called perindopril 4mg every day for the blood pressure.

History taking

(refer to OSCE set 1, station 1.12).

Initial approach

Greet the patient and introduce yourself by name, making sure you are talking to the right patient.

History of presenting complaint

Ask the patient what he knows about the operation and details of his presenting complaint. In this case his main problem is hearing loss in the left ear. You should ask about the cause for hearing loss and previous infection.

Always try to explore the reason for the proposed surgery and causes for the presenting pathology. In a patient presenting for a cataract operation, you should elicit the causes for a cataract. Diabetes mellitus or steroid use may be the cause of a cataract.

Past medical history

The patient may not volunteer the history of sarcoidosis since he is asymptomatic now. Certain past medical problems can only be elicited after asking specific questions during a system review. Therefore, a structured approach is more important. In this scenario, the patient may answer specific questions, such as did you have any chest problems in the past? Do you or did you suffer from shortness of breath or cough? Once you have elicited that the patient had sarcoidosis, you must ask further details on progression of the disease and treatment.

Sarcoidosis involves the eyes, bones, joints and heart (cardiomyopathy and conduction defect). It can also cause hypercalcaemic nephropathy and renal calculi. Active disease is treated with oral prednisolone and steroid eye drops.

Considering the patient's age you must ask the history of cardiovascular disease and cerebrovascular disease.

Key points

◆ Always follow a structured approach to gather information from the patient.
◆ Try to elicit the cause for the presenting surgical pathology.
◆ Remember to ask details on current and past medications.

Station 4.13 Simulation: post-induction hypotension

Information for the candidate

A 28-year-old female patient with diagnosis of a ruptured ectopic pregnancy is anaesthetised for a laparotomy.

On entering the station:

General anaesthesia was induced with etomidate and suxamethonium. The laryngoscopy view was grade 1 and the trachea has been intubated and ventilated. You are asked to take over the anaesthetic care soon after induction.

◆ Pre-operative BP: 110/84 mmHg, HR: 98 per minute, capillary refill: 4 seconds.

Soon after taking over, the monitor displays a heart rate of 110 and systolic blood pressure of 70 mm Hg.

Examiner's mark sheet

	marks	
Identifies hypotension.	2	☐
Checks the heart rate, saturation and $EtCO_2$.	2	☐
Increases inspired oxygen concentration.	2	☐
Rapidly infuses intravenous fluid.	2	☐
Continues volatile anaesthetic.	2	☐
Administers vasoconstrictors.	2	☐
Tilts the table.	2	☐

Informs the surgeon and asks for help.   2 ☐

Ensures that blood is available.   2 ☐

Manages this incident using a methodical approach.   2 ☐

| Total: | /20 |

Information for the examiner

Following pre-oxygenation, general anaesthesia was induced using a rapid sequence induction technique with etomidate and suxamethonium. The trachea was intubated and handed over to the candidate for further management of this patient. Soon after induction, the blood pressure decreases to 70 mm Hg and the heart rate increases to 110 per minute.

The monitor should display: HR: 110 per minute, BP: 70/30 mmHg, SaO_2: 96%, $EtCO_2$: 3.5 kPa and end-tidal isoflurane: 1.1%.

Hypotension following induction of general anaesthesia

A decrease in blood pressure is commonly observed after induction of general anaesthesia. This is due to vasodilatation and myocardial depression caused by most of the anaesthetic agents used at induction. In hypovolaemic patients, elderly patients and in patients with cardiovascular disease, a significant decrease in blood pressure is anticipated.

This patient was hypovolaemic prior to induction. On induction, vasodilatory and myocardial depressant effects of induction agents led to severe hypotension. There is also a possibility of ongoing blood loss. Immediate management includes measures to increase cardiac output and to maintain tissue perfusion. To control haemorrhage this patient needs immediate surgical intervention; therefore, in this situation it is advisable to proceed with the surgery.

Examiner's mark sheet

marks

Identify the problems in Figure 4.15a with regard to positioning of the patient   2 □

- The arm is hyperabducted.
- The neck is rotated to the other side.

What nerves are likely to be damaged in this position?   4 □

Both these factors related to positioning can cause traction on the brachial plexus. Rotation of the neck results in stretch of roots of the brachial plexus, particularly the upper nerve roots. This causes sensory loss over the outer aspect of the arm.

The ulnar nerve can be damaged at the elbow, behind the medial epicondyle (cubital groove).

What precautions would you take to avoid nerve damage?   5 □

- Head should be maintained in the neutral position.
- Arms should not be abducted >90°.
- Arms should be level with the shoulder.
- Elbows should be well padded.
- Forearm should be semipronated.

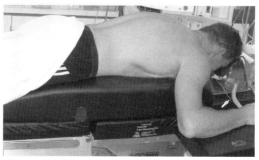

Figure 4.15b.

What nerves are likely to be damaged in the position shown in Figure 4.15b?   4

This patient is in the prone position. The nerves that are likely to be damaged are:

- Supra-orbital nerve.
- Infra-orbital nerve.
- Ulnar nerve at the elbow.
- Femoral nerve in the inguinal region.

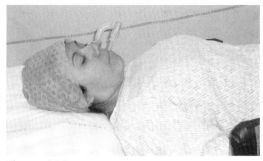

Figure 4.15c.

Identify the problems in Figure 4.15c   2

- The tracheal tube is not fixed and can be accidentally extubated.
- The eyes are not protected and are prone to damage.

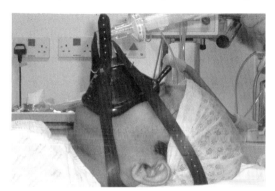

Figure 4.15d.

What nerve injuries can be expected in Figure 4.15d?   3 ☐

- The mask is pressing on the eye ball, which results in pressure on the optic nerve.
- Supra-orbital nerve damage results in ptosis.
- Damage to the buccal branch of the facial nerve results in drooping of the lip.

Total:	/20

Peripheral nerve injury

Seddon's classification is a scheme for describing nerve injury:

- Neurapraxia: pressure on the affected nerve with no loss of continuity.
- Axonotmesis: neural tube intact, but the axons are disrupted. These nerves are likely to recover.
- Neurotmesis: the neural tube is severed. These injuries are likely to be permanent without repair and will likely only achieve partial recovery at best.

Neurapraxia is concussion of the nerve, due to stretching or compression of the intact nerve fibres without any anatomical discontinuity of the fibres. Hence, there is complete recovery of sensory and motor function. Most cases recover in 6 weeks but it may be prolonged for up to 6 months.

Axonotmesis is rupture of the nerve fibres within an intact sheath. Initial clinical features resemble neurapraxia but the recovery of function is incomplete.

Neurotmesis is produced by either partial or complete division of the sheath and nerve fibre, which requires surgical treatment to restore function.

The usual mechanisms of nerve damage in an anaesthetised patient include stretch or compression. Peripheral nerves are subjected to compression between the bone and a hard surface, such as the operating table. Extreme positions of arms and limbs result in stretch of the nerves.

The brachial plexus is most vulnerable to damage as a result of positioning. The brachial plexus has a long, mobile and superficial course in the axilla, between points of fixation. The proximal point of fixation is the vertebral and prevertebral fascia, and the distal point of fixation is the axillary fascia. Rotation and extension of the neck, abduction, external rotation and extension of the arm cause stretching of the plexus. More often, upper roots of the brachial plexus (C5 and C6) are involved, resulting in Erb's palsy. The arm is internally rotated, the forearm is extended and the hand is pronated. Muscles paralysed are the deltoid, biceps, brachioradialis and supinator brevis. Involvement of lower roots (C8, T1) results in paralysis of small muscles of the hand and weakness of finger flexion (Klumpke's palsy). Sensory loss is observed over the inner aspect of the forearm and the medial three and a half fingers.

The ulnar nerve at the elbow is at risk of direct compression with any hard surface when the patient is supine with the arm pronated. Sensory loss is observed over the medial one and a half fingers and medial aspect of the palm. Flexor carpi ulnaris and the medial half of flexor digitorum profundus are paralysed, resulting in hyperextension of the little and ring fingers at the metacarpophalangeal joints. The patient cannot grip a piece of paper placed between the fingers due to paralysis of the small muscles of the hand. If the patient is asked to pinch a piece of paper between the thumb and the other fingers, the thumb assumes a fixed flexed position, as weakness of adductor pollicis brevis permits overaction of the long flexors of the thumb (refer to OSCE set 5, station 5.15, for peripheral nerve injury and resulting sensory loss).

The median nerve can be injured as a consequence of a prolonged tourniquet at the arm; the radial nerve can also be involved. This results in sensory loss over the thumb and medial two and a half fingers. The index finger and thumb cannot be flexed due to the paralysis of flexor carpi radialis and flexor pollicis longus. The muscles of the thenar eminence will be paralysed and wasted.

The radial nerve may be injured at the radial groove due to compression against the hard surface of an operating table. Sensory loss is observed over the dorsum of the forearm and dorsum of the thumb. Paralysis of extensors of the wrist and fingers results in wrist drop.

5. False. A shadow from a segment of the stomach is super-imposed on the heart shadow. In a loculated pericardial effusion the radiolucent shadow will lie on the periphery of the cardiac border.

6. True. Heartburn is one of the common symptoms of hiatus hernia.

7. True. An H_2 receptor antagonist, such as ranitidine, reduces hydrochloric acid production and reduces the pH of the gastric content.

8. False. Surgery can be performed as a day-case procedure, provided other criteria for day-case surgery are fulfilled.

9. False. This patient has an increased risk of aspiration; therefore, rapid sequence induction with tracheal intubation should be performed in this patient.

10. True. A barium meal or endoscopy is useful in assessing the size and severity of the hernia.

Hiatus hernia

Hiatus hernia occurs when a part of the stomach protrudes through the diaphragmatic hiatus into the thoracic cavity. A sliding hiatal hernia interferes with the normal anti-reflux mechanisms. As the lower oesophageal sphincter moves into the chest, the normal anatomical sphincter mechanism is lost. Therefore, regurgitation of gastric contents is more likely to occur. This also results in reflux oesophagitis.

In para-oesophageal hiatus hernia, a small part of the stomach rolls upwards into the chest through the hernia alongside the oesophagus. On an erect chest X-ray the hernia may be seen as a retrocardiac mass with or without an air-fluid level. The hernia is usually positioned to the left of the spine; however, larger hernias may extend beyond the cardiac confines and even mimic cardiomegaly.

Common symptoms include heartburn and water brush (acid taste in the mouth with reflex salivation) and dyspepsia. A barium meal or endoscopy should be performed to confirm the diagnosis. Retrosternal chest pain caused by reflux may sometimes mimic myocardial ischaemia.

Key points

◆ On an erect chest X-ray a hiatus hernia can be seen as a retrocardiac shadow.
◆ A hiatus hernia increases the risk of regurgitation of gastric contents.
◆ Appropriate measures should be taken to prevent regurgitation and aspiration of gastric contents.

Station 4.17 History taking: total hip replacement

Information for the candidate

In the following station you will be asked to take a history from a 70-year-old male patient who is scheduled to have a total hip replacement.

Examiner's mark sheet

	marks
Introduces him/herself to the patient and confirms that he/she is talking to the right person	1 ☐
Confirms the proposed surgery.	1 ☐
Enquires as to the reason for the proposed surgery.	1 ☐
Enquires about details of involvement of other joints.	1 ☐
Asks about neck pain and range of movement.	1 ☐
Elicits the impact on physical activity.	2 ☐

Examiner's mark sheet

                                                                        marks

Introduces him/herself and greets the patient.   1 ☐

Elicits the patient's concern about the epidural.   2 ☐

Asks details about previous epidural (duration, resiting).   2 ☐

Asks details about backache and any neurological problems.   2 ☐

Procedure

◆ After inserting the initial needle, a small thread-like tube is   2 ☐
   inserted into the epidural space, and then the needle is
   removed.
◆ A local anaesthetic (numbing medicine) infusion or a top   2 ☐
   up is given through a catheter to relieve the pain.
◆ There is a small risk of headache and it may cause a drop   2 ☐
   in blood pressure. The numbness and heavy legs will last
   for the duration of epidural analgesia.

Complications

◆ Effect of epidural on the progression of labour.   1 ☐
◆ Failure to provide complete analgesia.   2 ☐
◆ Failure of technique.   2 ☐

Uses clear language and avoids jargon.   1 ☐

Provides adequate reassurance, empathises and maintains   1 ☐
good eye contact.

Total:	/20

Information for the actor

You are 36 weeks pregnant. This is your second pregnancy. You had an epidural during your previous delivery; it was not successful. After 6 hours, another epidural was inserted, which worked but you delivered soon afterwards. Nobody explained to you why the first epidural failed.

This time you would like to have an epidural, but you are concerned that the same experience will happen again. You also suffer from backache. You are worried that it may get worse after having an epidural.

Technique of epidural anaesthesia

To obtain a patient's consent and co-operation, it may be useful for the patient to know the following information.

An intravenous cannula (a drip) is sited usually on the back of the hand and the procedure is performed with full aseptic precautions. The epidural is performed in the lateral or sitting position. The patient needs to keep still during the procedure and should indicate if they are experiencing pain or contractions. Fetal heart rate monitoring will be continued without interruption during the procedure.

First, numbing medicine is applied to the skin. Then, with a needle, the epidural space is located. A small tube, a catheter, is passed into the epidural space; the catheter should be secured well. Continuous infusion or intermittent top-ups of local anaesthetic are used to provide labour pain relief.

Epidural analgesia produces numbness and heaviness of the legs lasting for a few hours after the last top-up of the epidural. The possibility of global failure or missed segments should be explained. The anaesthetist or midwife will be checking the block. Blood pressure is checked at regular intervals. It usually takes about 15-20 minutes to provide pain relief after an initial dose. Occasionally, if the pain relief is incomplete, some adjustments of the dose and tube position (catheter may need to be withdrawn slightly) may be needed; rarely it has to be resited.

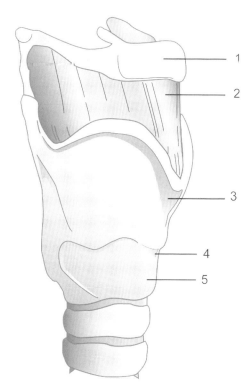

Figure 4.19a Lateral view of the larynx.

Name the parts labelled in Figure 4.19a

4 ☐

1. Hyoid bone.
2. Thyrohyoid membrane.
3. Thyroid cartilage.
4. Cricothyroid membrane.
5. Cricoid cartilage.

Total: /20

Information for the examiner

This patient is on the table, intravenous access is secured and standard monitoring is attached. The patient is now pre-oxygenated and is ready to be induced.

Cricoid pressure

Cricoid pressure was described by Sellick in 1961 to reduce the risk of aspiration syndrome. Correctly applied cricoid pressure occludes the oesophagus between the cricoid cartilage and cervical vertebra. The key to success of cricoid pressure is the proper application until the airway is protected using a cuffed tracheal tube. It is recommended to use 10N (1Kg) of pressure while the patient is awake and then to increase to 30N as the patient loses consciousness. More than 20N generally prevents passive aspiration and more than 40N may cause airway obstruction and a difficult laryngoscopy. Cricoid pressure can protect against aspiration, even in the presence of a nasogastric tube.

To identify the cricoid cartilage (refer to OSCE set 1, station 1.7), use the index finger to identify the thyroid notch and then follow the finger downwards in the midline; a dip is felt below the thyroid cartilage. This is the cricothyroid space. The prominent structure felt immediately below this is the cricoid cartilage. Once identified, it should be fixed between thumb and middle finger.

When applying the pressure, firm backward pressure is applied on the cricoid cartilage using the thumb and middle finger. The index finger should be placed on the thyroid cartilage to ensure that the cricoid ring is fixed in the midline position.

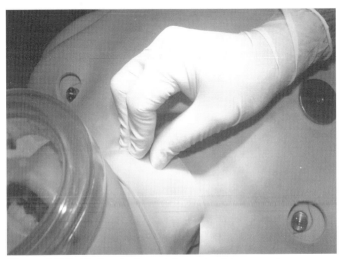

Figure 4.19b Method of applying cricoid pressure.

The appropriate technique and correct amount of pressure can be practised on cricoid pressure simulators. The amount of pressure required can be practised in pounds or kilogram weight on a weighing scale.

Key points

♦ The cricoid cartilage is a complete cartilaginous ring situated at the level of the 6th cervical vertebra in adults.
♦ Rapid sequence induction and the correct application of cricoid pressure reduces the risk of aspiration.

Station 4.20 Anatomy: caudal block

Information for the candidate

In the station you will be asked to demonstrate the technique of caudal block. A 6-year-old child weighing 20Kg is scheduled for an inguinal hernia repair.

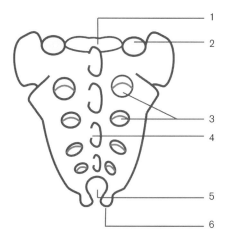

Figure 4.20 Posterior surface of the sacrum.

Examiner's mark sheet

marks

Name the structures labelled 1 to 3 on Figure 4.20   3 ☐

1. Sacral promontory.
2. Superior articular process.
3. Posterior sacral foramina.
4. Median crest.
5. Sacral hiatus.
6. Sacral cornu.

How is the sacral hiatus formed?   2 ☐

By failure of fusion of the 5th (occasionally the 4th as well) sacral laminar arch, resulting in a gap which is the sacral hiatus.

At what level do the spinal cord and dura end?   2 ☐

The spinal cord ends at the level of the L2 vertebra in children. The dura ends at the level of the S2 vertebra.

Describe the technique of performing a caudal block in this child   5 ☐

◆ Ensure that the patient (parent) has been consented.
◆ Ensure that venous access is secured.
◆ Under general anaesthesia.
◆ Aseptic technique.
◆ Lateral position.
◆ Identify the sacral hiatus.
◆ 22G needle or cannula introduced at a 45° angle to the skin.
◆ Puncture the sacro-coccygeal membrane.
◆ Flatten the needle and advance 1-2cm.
◆ Stabilise the needle.
◆ Negative aspiration.
◆ Inject the local anaesthetic. 12-16ml of 0.25% bupivacaine can be used in this patient (maximum 2mg/Kg of bupivacaine, ropivacaine or levobupivacaine).

What volume would you use in adults?   2 ▢

20-30ml of 0.25% to 0.5% of bupivacaine is used in adults.

What are the benefits of caudal block in this child?   2 ▢

It supplements general anaesthesia and provides both intra-operative and postoperative analgesia.

What are the complications of caudal block?   4 ▢

Bleeding, intravascular injection, subarachnoid injection, inadequate analgesia, failure of the technique.

Total:	/20

Anatomy of the caudal epidural space

The sacrum is a large triangular bone. The apex articulates with the coccyx and the base articulates with the 5th lumbar vertebra. On the dorsal surface of the sacrum in the midline is the middle sacral crest, surmounted by 3 or 4 tubercles, the rudimentary spinous processes of the upper 3 or 4 sacral vertebrae. The laminae of the 5th sacral vertebra, and sometimes those of the 4th, fail to meet and thus a deficiency occurs in the posterior wall of the sacral canal. This is called the sacral hiatus. The tubercles which represent the inferior articular processes of the 5th sacral vertebra are named the sacral cornua. The sacral hiatus is covered by a sacro-coccygeal membrane. The sacral canal contains areolar connective tissue, fat, sacral nerves, lymphatics, the filum terminale and a rich venous plexus.

Caudal block

In children, caudal block is generally performed after inducing general anaesthesia. Important landmarks to be identified are the sacral hiatus and the two posterior superior iliac spines which form an equilateral triangle. The sacral cornua are felt on either side of the hiatus. Under aseptic technique, a 20 or 22G needle or cannula is inserted through the sacral hiatus in a slightly cranial direction to pierce the sacrococcygeal membrane. A click is felt as the needle passes through the membrane. Because of rich vascularity and the possibility of anatomical variation in attachment of the dura, the need for careful negative aspiration cannot be overomphasized. After negative aspiration, the calculated mixture of local anaesthetic should be injected slowly. At times, ketamine (at a dose of 0.5mg/Kg body weight) is added in the mixture to improve the quality and duration of postoperative analgesia. In view of the technical ease involved and relatively free epidural space with minimal fat, a catheter can be introduced upwards to provide analgesia even for upper abdominal and thoracic procedures.

The volume of 0.25% bupivacaine or levobupivacaine used depends on the site of surgical procedure:

- Lumbosacral block - 0.5ml/Kg.
- Thoracolumbar block - 1.0ml/Kg.
- Mid-thoracic block - 1.25ml/Kg.

As the maximum dose of bupivacaine is 2mg/Kg, to make up the volume 0.9% saline can be added.

Key points

- A caudal epidural is an important regional technique used to provide intra-operative and postoperative analgesia in paediatric surgery.
- Adjuncts such as clonidine or ketamine are added to the mixture to improve quality and duration of analgesia.
- In view of vascularity, inadvertent intravascular injection and local anaesthetic toxicity are possible.

OSCE
set 5

Station 5.1 Anaesthetic equipment: airway equipment

Information for the candidate

In this station you will be shown some photographs of airway equipment and asked further questions related to tracheal intubation.

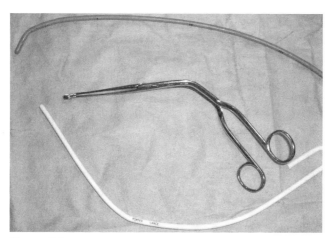

Figure 5.1a.

Examiner's mark sheet

marks

Name the equipment in Figure 5.1a 3 ☐

* Gum elastic bougie (Eschmann tracheal tube introducer).
* Magill's forceps.
* Intubating stylet.

What are Magill's forceps used for?   2 ☐

Magill's forceps are used as an aid for nasotracheal intubation, to insert a throat pack, to pass a nasogastric tube and to remove a foreign body from the oropharynx.

What is the bougie used for?   1 ☐

It is used as an aid in difficult intubation to facilitate tracheal intubation.

How would you grade the laryngoscopic view?   4 ☐

Cormack and Lehane's classification of laryngoscopic view:

- Grade 1: most of the glottis is seen.
- Grade 2: only the posterior part of the glottis is seen.
- Grade 3: only the epiglottis is visible.
- Grade 4: even the epiglottis is not visible.

What manoeuvres are useful in improving the   3 ☐
laryngoscopic view?

- Optimum sniffing position.
- BURP: backward, upward, right-ward pressure on the thyroid cartilage.
- In rapid sequence induction, excessive force applied during cricoid pressure may worsen the laryngoscopic view; a transient release of cricoid pressure may improve the laryngoscopic view.

What signs would indicate that the bougie is in the   2 ☐
trachea rather than in the oesophagus?

When the angled tip of the bougie slides down the trachea, the tracheal rings can be felt as clicks. A distal hold up is sensed as a slight resistance when the tip enters the bronchial tree. If the patient is not fully paralysed, the patient is likely to cough as the bougie enters the trachea.

What are the complications of using a bougie? 2

Insertion of a bougie can be associated with complications, such as soft tissue trauma and bronchial rupture.

What should you do if the bougie is in the correct 1 place, but the tube is caught at the laryngeal inlet?

A 90° anticlockwise rotation of the tube facilitates passage of the tube into the trachea.

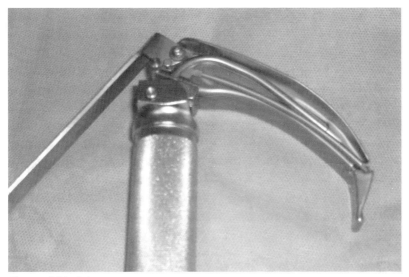

Figure 5.1b A laryngoscope.

Name the laryngoscope in Figure 5.1b and state its 2 clinical use

The McCoy laryngoscope is a levering laryngoscope. The blade has a tip which when levered lifts the epiglottis and can convert Cormack and Lehane's grade 3 view into a grade 2 or a grade 2 into a grade 1 view.

Total: /20

Key points

◆ A gum elastic bougie is a useful device in managing difficult intubation. It is more effective than an intubating stylet when the laryngoscopic view is grade 3.
◆ A McCoy laryngoscope has a levering tip which moves anteriorly and lifts the epiglottis.

Station 5.2 Data interpretation: lung function tests

Information for the candidate

A 62-year-old male patient is scheduled for total hip replacement. He has smoked 10-15 cigarettes per day for the past 30 years. He also gives a history of shortness of breath and cough. Table 5.2a shows the results of lung function tests performed during the pre-operative assessment.

Table 5.2a Results of lung function tests.

Spirometry Age: 62 years, Height: 170cm, Weight: 68Kg, Sex: male.

	Predicted value	Observed value Pre	% pred	Observed value Post	% pred
FVC L	3.8	3.4	89	3.3	87
FEV1 L	2.9	1.8	62	1.9	66
FEV1/FVC %	76	55	-	58	-
FEF 25-75 L/S	2.8	1.2	43	-	-
PEFR L/S	7.5	3.5	47	3.8	51

Lung volumes

	Predicted value	Observed value	% pred
FRC L	2.7	4.2	156%
VC L	3.8	3.5	92%
RV L	2.1	3.2	152%
TLC L	6.2	7.2	116%

Pre: prior to bronchodilator therapy
Post: after bronchodilator therapy

Examiner's mark sheet

Please tick the correct answer - true or false.   **marks**

1. These results are compatible with restrictive lung   True False 2 ☐
   disease
2. The FEV1 is normal for this patient.   True False 2 ☐
3. This patient is likely to have emphysema.   True False 2 ☐
4. The FVC is the volume of air breathed out in the   True False 2 ☐
   first second during forced expiration.
5. The most common cause is acute asthma.   True False 2 ☐
6. Bronchodilators are useful in this patient.   True False 2 ☐
7. The FRC can be measured using spirometry.   True False 2 ☐
8. The ECG may show abnormal P waves.   True False 2 ☐
9. This patient may benefit from steroids.   True False 2 ☐
10. Carbon monoxide transfer would be increased in   True False 2 ☐
    this patient.

Total: /20

Answers

1. False. The FVC is normal and FEV1 is markedly reduced in this patient. The ratio of FEV1/FVC is reduced, suggestive of obstructive lung disease. In restrictive lung disease, the FVC would be reduced and the ratio of FEV1/FVC would be increased or may remain normal.

2. False. The FEV1 is reduced. It is 62% of actual predicted value.

3. True. Increased total lung capacity (TLC) and increased residual volume (RV) suggest emphysema.

4. False. Forced expiratory volume in 1 second (FEV1) is the volume of air breathed out in the first second, whereas forced vital capacity (FVC) is the volume of air breathed out during forced expiration following a deep inspiration.

5. False. Asthma is a reversible obstructive airway disease which improves with bronchodilator therapy, therefore post-test results should show more than a 15% increase in the FEV1 value.

6. False. The test shows no significant improvement in results following administration of bronchodilators.

7. False. The functional residual capacity (FRC) can be measured using a nitrogen wash-out or helium dilution technique.

8. True. As a result of obstructive airway disease, the resulting hypoxic pulmonary vasoconstriction can lead to cor pulmonale. Tall and wide P waves are seen in right atrial enlargement secondary to cor pulmonale.

9. True. In COAD, a trial of inhaled steroids are given; if they are found to be of benefit in reducing the symptoms then they are continued; otherwise they are cautiously withdrawn.

10. False. Carbon monoxide transfer is reduced in emphysema.

Lung function tests

This patient's lung function tests are suggestive of obstructive airway disease. Measured FEV1 is markedly reduced; the ratio of FEV1/FVC is 55%. Lung volumes suggest hyperinflation (raised TLC) and gas trapping (raised RV).

Lung function tests are interpreted by comparing the observed values with predicted values. Predicted values depend on the patient's age, sex and height. Spirometry is the simplest of all the lung function tests. It is a measure of airflow and lung volumes during forced expiration following a full inspiration. FEV1, FVC and the ratio of FEV1/FVC are the 3 basic measurements obtained from spirometry. These 3 parameters are useful in distinguishing obstructive lung disease from restrictive lung disease.

In obstructive airway disease (asthma and COAD), airflow during expiration is reduced resulting in a reduced FEV1. A FEV1/FVC ratio less than 70% indicates obstructive airway disease; the FEV1 indicates the severity of airway obstruction. In severe obstructive airway disease, FEV1 is less than 40% of the predicted value.

In restrictive airway disease, FVC is reduced; the absolute value of FEV1 is less than predicted, but the ratio of FEV1/FVC is normal or may be high. Restrictive disorders are caused by reduced compliance of the chest wall (obesity, kyphoscoliosis) or by interstitial lung fibrosis.

The above is summarised in Table 5.2b.

Table 5.2b Lung function tests.		
Test	**Restrictive lung disease**	**Obstructive lung disease**
FEV1	Reduced	Reduced
FVC	Reduced	Normal/Increased
FEV1 / FVC	Normal/Increased	Decreased

A forced expiratory flow between 25-75% of the FVC (maximum mid-expiratory flow) can also be obtained from spirometry, indicating airflow in medium and small airways. It is reduced in asthma.

To assess the reversibility of airway obstruction, spirometry is repeated 15-30 minutes after bronchodilator therapy. An improvement of 15% of FEV1 or FVC is considered as significant reversibility. A significant improvement in spirometry following bronchodilator therapy suggests asthma. Airflow obstruction in COAD is irreversible.

The carbon monoxide transfer factor (TLCO) is the product of the two primary measurements during breathholding: the CO transfer coefficient (KCO) and the alveolar volume (VA).

Because of a non-linear increase in pulmonary capillary oxygen tension, calculation of the transfer factor for oxygen is difficult. Carbon monoxide is a gas with 230 times more affinity for haemoglobin when compared to that of oxygen. The calculation of TLCO is based on the assumption that plasma CO tension is negligible. Several methods have been developed to measure TLCO, the commonly used ones being single breath (gold standard), and multiple breath tests. The values are expressed as mmol/min/kPa. The size of TLCO will depend on a variety of parameters, including the amount of available haemoglobin, the volume of ventilated alveoli and perfused lung capillaries, and their relation to each other. Values for TLCO decrease with age and increase with physical activity and increased lung volumes. A decreased TLCO will be found in both restrictive and obstructive lung disorders.

Key points

◆ A reduced FEV1 with a reduced FEV1/FVC ratio suggests obstructive airway disease.
◆ A reduced FVC with a normal or high FEV1/FVC ratio suggests restrictive lung disease.
◆ An increase in FVC or FEV1 by more than 15% following bronchodilators suggests significant reversibility.

Station 5.3 Data interpretation: statistics

Information for the candidate

In this station you will be provided with a set of statistical data. Read the given data and answer the questions as true or false on the marking sheet.

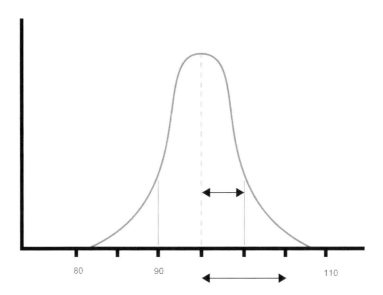

Figure 5.3a Represents the heart rate of 100 ASA 1 children on admission to a day-surgery unit (x axis: heart rate, y axis: number of children).

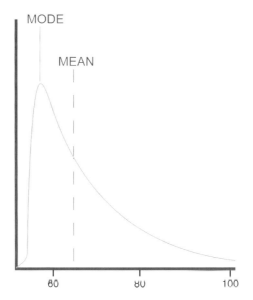

Figure 5.3b Represents the heart rate of 100 patients (age varying from 30-70 years and ASA 1-4) 5 minutes after administration of 1.5µg/Kg of fentanyl (x axis: heart rate, y axis: number of patients).

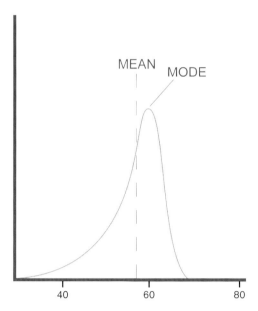

Figure 5.3c Represents the heart rate of 100 hypertensive patients 2 weeks after starting a new beta blocker (x axis: heart rate, y axis: number of patients).

Examiner's mark sheet

Please tick the correct answer - true or false.   *marks*

1. Figure 5.3a represents a Gaussian distribution of   True False 2 ☐
    data.
2. Parametric tests can be used for the data in Figure   True False 2 ☐
    5.3a.
3. In Figure 5.3a, the mean is usually greater than the   True False 2 ☐
    median.
4. Figure 5.3a also represents a positively skewed   True False 2 ☐
    distribution.
5. In Figure 5.3a, 95% of the observations fall within   True False 2 ☐
    one SD.
6. In Figure 5.3b, data are normally distributed.   True False 2 ☐

7. In Figure 5.3c, data are negatively skewed.   True False 2 ☐
8. A student's t-test may be used to compare the True False 2 ☐
   parametric data.
9. A Chi-square test is used for analysing the True False 2 ☐
   qualitative data.
10. A p<0.01 means that the results are significant at True False 2 ☐
   the 5% level.

Total: /20

Answers

1. True. This is a symmetrical bell-shaped distribution where mean, median and mode are all equal. In quantitative data, variation is expressed around the central tendency.

2. True.

3. False. As explained in 1 above.

4. False. This represents a normal distribution.

5. False. In a normal distribution, 68% of the observations fall within one standard deviation (SD). 95% of the observations fall within two SD and 99.7% of the observations fall within three SD.

6. False. It is positively skewed; distribution is not symmetric. It has a longer tail towards higher values. In general, in a skewed distribution, the median and interquartile range are more appropriate.

7. True. It has a longer tail towards lower values.

8. True. A student's t-test may be used to compare two sets of normally distributed data. If the two sets of data belong to the same group of patients, a paired t-test is used. A set of blood pressure readings before/after administering propofol can be compared using a paired t-test. Two separate series of results can be compared using an unpaired t-test.

9. True.

10. False. It means that the results are significant at the 1% level.

Statistical values

In many physiological measurements the shape of frequency distribution approaches the normal distribution curve. The central location can be described by a mean which is the same as the mode and median. The variability from the central location is described in terms of standard deviation. A normal distribution has the characteristic bell curve. In a normal distribution, 68% of all observations fall within a range of +/-1 standard deviation, 95% within +/-2 standard deviation and 99.99% within +/-4 standard deviation.

When the frequency distribution curve is not symmetrical, the distribution is skewed. In a skewed distribution mean, the median and mode have different values. If one of the values or observations increases, the mean of the sample increases without changing the mode and median. The standard deviation will have a large value, usually more than half the mean in a skewed distribution. The variability of values is better described by percentiles (interquartile range). The difference between the first and third quartiles is known as the interquartile range.

In a positive skew, the mode is at the top of the curve, the median is higher than that, and the mean is higher than the median. In a negative skew, the mode is at the top of the curve, the median is lower than it, and the mean is lower than the median.

Key points

◆ A normal distribution has the characteristic bell curve.
◆ In a normal distribution, the mean, median and mode all have the same value.
◆ In a normal distribution, variability is described in terms of standard deviation.

Station 5.4 Data interpretation: arterial blood gas result

Information for the candidate

In this station you will be presented with a set of arterial blood gas results. Read the results and answer the questions as true or false.

A 76-year-old lady, with a weight of 50Kg, undergoing intra-medullary nailing of the femur developed ST segment depression and a few ventricular ectopics, and sustained a cardiac arrest. Following intense resuscitation for 5 minutes, cardiac output was established. Her blood pressure is now 90/50 mmHg and HR is 130/minute. A set of blood results obtained at this stage has been listed below in Table 5.4 (she is ventilated with a FiO_2 of 0.5). Her past medical history includes hypertension and ischaemic heart disease.

Table 5.4 Blood gas results.		
pH: 7.19	PCO_2: 4.8 kPa	PO_2: 20 kPa
BE: -12.1mmol/L	tCO_2: 11mmol/L	HCO_3^-: 10mmol/L
Na^+: 140mmol/L	K^+: 3.0mmol/L	Hb: 5.0g/dL
SaO_2: 100%	Cl^-: 110mmol/L	

Examiner's mark sheet

Please tick the correct answer - true or false.   **marks**

1. The above results show metabolic acidosis.   True False 2 ☐
2. There is compensatory respiratory alkalosis.   True False 2 ☐
3. The anion gap is increased.   True False 2 ☐
4. The cause of cardiac arrest could be fat   True False 2 ☐
   embolism.
5. 150mmol of sodium bicarbonate should be   True False 2 ☐
   given immediately.
6. Hypokalaemia in this patient can be due to   True False 2 ☐
   acidosis.

7. This patient needs a blood transfusion.   True   False   2 ☐
8. The standard bicarbonate value is directly   True   False   2 ☐
   measured by a blood gas analyser.
9. The base excess in this sample is calculated   True   False   2 ☐
   by adding base to the blood sample to
   restore the normal pH.
10. Arterial oxygen content is about 12ml/100ml.   True   False   2 ☐

Total:	/20

Answers

1. True. The pH suggests acidosis. The bicarbonate level is markedly low and PCO_2 is within normal limits.

2. False. This blood gas result is suggestive of primary metabolic acidosis without any metabolic compensation. Compensation to metabolic acidosis is achieved by hyperventilation which lowers the PCO_2.

3. True. The normal anion gap is 12-18, which can be calculated as $(Na^+ + K^+) - (HCO_3^- + Cl^-)$; $(140 + 3 - 10 + 110) = 23$.

4. True. As this patient is undergoing intra-medullary nailing of the femur, fat embolism could be possible. Another possible cause of cardiac arrest in this patient could be a massive pulmonary embolism.

5. False. Sodium bicarbonate should be administered if the pH is less than 7.1. There are several disadvantages to administering sodium bicarbonate. Sodium bicarbonate is converted into CO_2 which may cause further acidosis. $NaHCO_3^-$ administration results in extracellular alkalosis, with a resulting shift of the oxygen dissociation curve to the left which reduces oxygen delivery to the tissues.

6. False. In acidosis, extracellular H^+ concentration is increased; H^+ enters the cell and potassium ions move out of the cells resulting in hyperkalaemia.

7. True. This patient has a low haemoglobin and hence needs a blood transfusion, which would improve oxygen delivery to the tissues, including the myocardium.

8. False. The blood gas analyser directly measures pO_2, pCO_2, and pH. The actual bicarbonate, standard bicarbonate, and base excess are calculated from the pH and pCO_2 using the Siggard-Anderson normogram.

9. False. Although that is the definition of a base excess, in this sample it is calculated as described above in 8.

10. False. It is 6.7ml/100ml.

Interpretation of blood gas results

Arterial blood gas interpretation should be considered in conjunction with the patient's clinical history:

◆ The first step is to determine whether there is an acid base disorder. First read the pH; a normal value is 7.36-7.44; a pH lower than 7.36 suggests acidosis and a pH more than 7.44 suggests alkalosis.
◆ The second step is to determine the primary acid base disorder. The primary acid base disorder will go in the same direction of pH. The compensatory mechanism will not overcorrect the primary disorder. Then read the $PaCO_2$ and bicarbonate values. An abnormal $PaCO_2$ value (normal $PaCO_2$ is 4.6-5.6kPa) indicates a respiratory disorder and an abnormal bicarbonate value (normal is 22-26mmol/L) indicates a metabolic disorder.
◆ The next step is to determine the compensatory mechanism. The compensatory mechanism will bring the pH back towards normal but will not overcorrect. In the given sample, the pH and bicarbonate are low; hence, metabolic acidosis is the primary disorder. The $PaCO_2$ value is normal and hence there is no respiratory compensation. Metabolic acidosis is compensated by hyperventilation, which by lowering $PaCO_2$, increases the pH.
◆ The standard base excess is the amount of acid or alkali required to restore the normal pH at a PCO_2 of 5.3kPa and temperature of 37°C.

Describe the origin of the sciatic nerve and its relations in the gluteal region   4

The sciatic nerve is formed by the fusion of two nerve trunks. The tibial component is formed from the anterior branches of the ventral rami of L4, 5 and S1, 2, 3 nerve roots. The peroneal component is formed from the posterior branches of the same nerve roots. It enters the gluteal region through the greater sciatic foramen below the piriformis muscle. In the gluteal region, it lies anterior to the gluteus maximus muscle and posterior to the obturator internus and quadratus femoris muscles. Here the nerve is approximately at the midpoint between the ischial tuberosity and the greater trochanter. It continues downward along the posteromedial aspect of the femur. At the apex of the popliteal fossa it divides into the tibial and common peroneal nerves.

Name the various approaches to blocking the sciatic nerve   2

There are several approaches to blocking the sciatic nerve. These include a posterior (Labat's), anterior, lateral and inferior approach in the supine lithotomy position.

Describe the technique of sciatic nerve block using the classic posterior approach   3

- Position: lateral with the side to be blocked uppermost.
- Landmarks: posterior superior iliac spine (PSIS) and the greater trochanter (GT).
- A straight line is drawn from the PSIS to the upper border of the GT. From the midpoint of this line a perpendicular line is drawn caudally.
- Needle insertion: 5cm from the midpoint, along the perpendicular line, the needle is inserted perpendicular to the skin in all planes (this point will lie on the line joining the sacral hiatus and the GT).

What is the desired motor response after placement of the stimulator needle, while performing a sciatic nerve block?　　2　☐

When the tibial component is stimulated, plantar flexion of the foot or toes is observed, stimulation of the peroneal component results in dorsiflexion or eversion of the foot.

How much local anaesthetic is required for an effective block?　　1　☐

10-20ml of 0.25-0.5% bupivacaine or L-bupivacaine or, 1% lidocaine/prilocaine

Total:	/20

Sciatic nerve block

Sciatic nerve blocks can be used for anaesthesia of the skin of the posterior aspect of the thigh, the leg below the level of the knee (except the medial aspect of the leg which is supplied by the saphenous nerve), and the hip and knee joint.

The gluteal approach to blocking the sciatic nerve is already described above. The posterior subgluteal approach is between the ischial tuberosity medially and GT laterally.

The sciatic nerve divides into peroneal and tibial components approximately 5-7cm above the popliteal crease in the apex of the popliteal fossa, although this can be variable. The nerve can be blocked at this level either through the posterior or lateral approach. In the posterior approach, at the apex of the popliteal fossa, between the semitendinosus muscle medially and biceps femoris muscle laterally, the needle is introduced. The nerve lies lateral to the popliteal artery pulsation. In the lateral approach, the needle is passed between the tendons of vastus lateralis and biceps (intertendinous approach).

Key points

- Be honest.
- Apologize if there is a genuine mistake, but do not waste time in being too apologetic throughout the session. No matter how sorry you feel, you will only receive the assigned 1 or 2 marks.
- It is good practice to discuss this risk pre-operatively in susceptible cases and mention about the discussion during counselling.
- Explain that in a difficult airway and in an emergency, the priority is to secure the airway rather than avoiding dental trauma.
- Describe the importance of inserting the tube into a windpipe in time to avoid hypoxia.
- Preserve the dislodged tooth.
- Inform the consultant and document it in the notes.
- Give attention to pain relief, secondary to dental injury.
- Involve the hospital dentist.
- Send a difficult airway alert to the patient, document it in the anaesthesia record and send a letter to the family physician.
- Have a sympathetic voice throughout the session, however annoying the actor is.

Station 5.7 Technical skill: chest drain insertion

Information for the candidate

You have anaesthetised a patient for a laparoscopic cholecystectomy. This patient is known to have COAD with mild emphysematous changes in the chest X-ray. Half way through the procedure the patient's saturation decreased to 90%. Increasing inspired oxygen to 100% and hand ventilating failed to increase the saturation. Other vital parameters are: BP: 85/50 mm Hg, heart rate: 110/minute, peak airway pressure: 30 mmHg. On auscultation there is reduced air entry on the right side. You will be asked questions on the further management of this patient.

Examiner's mark sheet

marks

This patient's saturation is 90% on 100% oxygen and is most likely to have a tension pneumothorax on the right side

What is your immediate management?

2 ☐

Needle thoracocentesis.

How would you perform the procedure? Indicate the landmarks (on a manikin or actor)

2 ☐

Identify the 2nd intercostal space in the mid-clavicular line and insert a 14G wide-bore cannula (venflon) into the intercostal space, remove the needle, leaving the cannula in place.

How would you locate the 2nd intercostal space?

1 ☐

Feel for the sternal angle which corresponds to the 2nd rib and the space below it is the 2nd intercostal space.

On insertion of the cannula there is a sudden escape of air and now the oxygen saturation is 96%

What would you do next?

2 ☐

A chest drain should be inserted.

How would you insert the chest drain? Indicate the landmarks

2 x 5* ☐
=10

- Choose the correct site; 5th intercostal space on the right side, between the mid-axillary and anterior axillary line*.
- Clean the area with an antiseptic solution and apply a sterile drape.

◆ Make a 2-3cm horizontal incision on the upper border of the lower rib*.
◆ Use blunt dissection with an artery clamp and finger*.
◆ Puncture the pleura using a blunt artery clamp guided by the finger.
◆ Insert a finger to sweep the lung away from the pleura.
◆ Clamp the proximal end of the chest tube and advance the tube into the pleural cavity.
◆ Connect the tube to the underwater seal drainage and release the clamp*.
◆ Suture the tube to the chest wall and apply a dressing.
◆ Obtain a chest X-ray*.

What are the complications of chest drain insertion? State three complications

3

◆ Visceral injury: laceration of the lung, liver, pericardium and heart.
◆ Injury to intercostal vessels and nerves.
◆ Haemothorax.
◆ Subcutaneous emphysema.
◆ Infection.
◆ Incorrect tube position, kinking of the tube and tube blockage.

Total: /20

Tension pneumothorax

The objective of this station is to assess the knowledge and skill that is essential for diagnosing and treating a tension pneumothorax (a critical incident during the intra-operative period). This station can also be simulated on a simulator.

◆ Tension pneumothorax is a life-threatening emergency and can result in cardiorespiratory arrest.
◆ Prompt diagnosis and immediate treatment is essential.

Management of suspected pneumothorax

- Turn off the nitrous oxide and administer 100% oxygen.
- Confirm diagnosis of pneumothorax:
  - auscultate both sides of the chest;
  - percuss the chest for hyper resonance;
  - feel for tracheal deviation;
  - rule out other causes of high airway pressure.
- If significant hypotension is present, a tension pneumothorax should be considered.

Treatment of tension pneumothorax

- Circulatory support with intravenous fluid and vasopressor drugs.
- Decompress the pneumothorax by inserting a large bore intravenous cannula at the 2nd intercostal space in the mid-clavicular line.
- Once the intrathoracic pressure is reduced, venous return increases, which increases cardiac output and improves gas exchange.

A chest drain must be inserted following needle thoracocentesis.

Insertion of a chest drain

A chest drain is usually inserted at the 5th intercostal space between the mid-axillary and anterior axillary line. The skin should be incised over the upper border of the lower rib to avoid injury to the neurovascular bundle which runs along the inner aspect of the lower border of the rib. Although a rigid trochar is provided along with the chest drain tube, it should be avoided as it increases the likelihood of injury to the lung. After incising the skin and deep tissues, blunt dissection is achieved using artery forceps. Once the pleura is punctured, a finger tip should be inserted to sweep the lung away from the insertion site. Chest drain tubes of size 20-28 FG (French Gauge) are suitable for most adults. These tubes have side holes to facilitate drainage and a radio-opaque line so that the position can be checked using chest X-ray.

The position of the tip of the tube should be aimed at the apex for draining air and towards the base of the lung for draining fluid. The chest tube should be attached to a drainage system which allows one direction of flow (from the patient to the drainage system), an underwater seal device. One-way flutter valves may also be used (Heimlich valve), which allow earlier mobilisation and the potential for an earlier discharge of patients with a chest drain.

The chest drain should not be removed until bubbling has ceased and the chest X-ray demonstrates re-inflation of the lung. The chest drain should be removed either while the patient performs a Valsalva manoeuvre or during the expiratory phase.

The underwater seal device should have the following features (Figure 5.7):

◆ The tube connecting the chest drain should have minimum resistance.
◆ The tube should be approximately 3cm below the surface of the water. If it is more than 5cm it increases the resistance for the air or fluid to escape from the pleural cavity.
◆ The bottle should be at least 45cm below the level of the patient's chest. Water may be drawn into the pleural cavity during maximal negative inspiratory effort if it is more close to the patient.

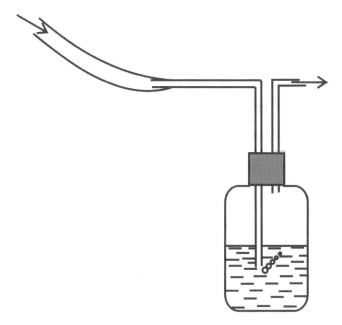

Figure 5.7 Single bottle chest drainage system.

The chest drain bottle should always be kept below the level of the patient. If suction is required a low pressure high volume suction (-10 to -20cmH$_2$O) should be used. It is used only for a non-resolving pneumothorax.

Key points

◆ Tension pneumothorax results in impaired gas exchange and severe hypotension.
◆ Treatment includes immediate needle thoracocentesis followed by insertion of a chest drain.
◆ A chest X-ray should be performed after insertion of the chest drain.
◆ Respiratory swing in the fluid in the chest tube is useful in assessing tube patency.

Station 5.8 Clinical examination: arterial and venous pulses, and pressures

Information for the candidate

In this station you will be asked to perform a clinical examination to check the arterial and venous pulses, and to assess arterial and venous pressures.

Examiner's mark sheet

marks

Introduces him/herself to the patient.	1 ☐
Feels radial pulses on both sides.	2 ☐
Correctly elicits the rate and rhythm.	2 ☐
Looks for a collapsing pulse.	2 ☐

Feels for the brachial and carotid pulse, and listens for carotid bruits.   3 ☐

Correctly measures the blood pressure (values +/- 10 mmHg of the examiner's reading).   2 ☐

Measures or mentions that he/she will measure this on both sides.   2 ☐

Uses the correct method of examining the jugular venous pulse.   2 ☐

How would you measure the height of the jugular venous pulse?   2 ☐

Determine the upper level of the JVP and measure the vertical distance between this point and the sternal angle.

How would you differentiate between the JVP and carotid pulse?   2 ☐

The JVP has a definite upper level and becomes more prominent with hepatojugular reflex; the carotid pulse is easily palpable.

Total: /20

Jugular venous pulse

The internal jugular vein is directly connected to the superior vena cava and right heart without any intervening valves.

The jugular venous pulse (JVP) provides information about venous return and right heart function. The patient is examined in a semi-recumbent position at 45° with their head supported on a pillow. The internal jugular vein runs downwards from a point below the ear lobe, above and behind the angle of the mandible, between the two heads of the sternocleidomastoid muscle to join the subclavian vein behind the sternoclavicular joint. The measurement of the JVP is expressed as the vertical distance from the manubriosternal angle to the maximum height of pulsations in the internal jugular vein. It is normally less than 3cm. This equates to a right atrial pressure of 8cm of water, as in this position, the manubriosternal angle is about 5cm above the centre of the right atrium. The pulsations are better visualised than felt. The complex waveforms (a, c, x, y) and the changes with respiration and compression on the liver differentiates it from the carotid pulse.

Differentiation of the JVP from the carotid pulse

- The JVP has a definitive upper level (in a normal healthy person it is <4cm).
- The JVP is multiphasic: it has 2 positive waves, a and v. The carotids have a single beat.
- The JVP is better seen; the carotids are better felt.
- The JVP is easily occluded.
- The JVP varies with the angle of the neck; the carotids remain stable.
- The JVP varies with respiration; the pressure falls with inspiration.
- There is a positive hepatojugular reflex with the JVP. On pressing the right subcostal (liver) area there is a transient elevation of the JVP.

Peripheral pulses

The radial pulse is used for assessing the rhythm and heart rate. Both radial pulses should be felt simultaneously to compare the volume and timing. Stenosis of the subclavian artery results in a low volume radial pulse on the affected side. Radiofemoral delay is observed in coarctation of the aorta.

The brachial pulse is used for assessing the character of the pulse. In a hypotensive patient and with peripheral vasoconstriction all peripheral pulses may be feeble. The carotid pulse is the most central pulse and is better for assessing the character.

Key points

- Use an organised approach to examine the peripheral pulses.
- A slow rising pulse is seen in severe aortic stenosis.
- Radiofemoral delay is seen in coarctation of the aorta.
- A collapsing pulse is seen in aortic regurgitation and a hyperdynamic circulation.
- Look for the jugular venous pulse in a semi-recumbent position at 45°.

Station 5.9 Measuring equipment: Severinghaus carbon dioxide electrode

Information for the candidate

In this station you will be asked questions on CO_2 measurement, to assess your knowledge of clinical measurement.

Examiner's mark sheet

marks

State how you would measure $PaCO_2$ from a given blood sample   2 ☐

Using a Severinghaus CO_2 electrode.

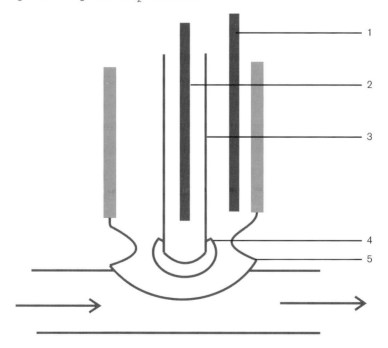

Figure 5.9 Severinghaus electrode.

Name the parts labelled 1, 2 and 3 in Figure 5.9   3

1. Reference electrode.
2. H^+ sensitive glass electrode.
3. H^+ sensitive glass.
4. Bicarbonate-containing nylon mesh.
5. CO_2 permeable membrane.

What is the principle involved measuring PCO_2 using this electrode?   2

CO_2 reacts with water to produce carbonic acid which then dissociates into hydrogen and bicarbonate ions. H^+ ions generated are proportional to the concentration of CO_2. The potential developed across the H^+ sensitive glass electrode is measured by a voltmeter.

How would you calibrate a CO_2 electrode?   2

It is calibrated by equilibrating the buffer using standard solutions containing known CO_2 concentrations to establish the relationship between pH and CO_2.

What methods are available for measuring CO_2 in a gas mixture?   4

CO_2 concentration in a gas mixture can be measured using mass spectrometry, Raman spectrometry, an infrared analyser and gas chromatography.

What is the principle of an infrared analyser?   2

Gases containing two or more dissimilar atoms absorb infrared radiation. By measuring the fraction of radiation of a known wavelength absorbed by the gas mixture, the partial pressure of a particular gas can be determined.

At what wavelength does CO_2 absorb infrared light?   1 ☐

CO_2 absorbs infrared light at 4.3μm.

What are the sources of error in an infrared analyser?   4 ☐

◆ There is overlap in the absorption wavelengths of different gases. Presence of other gases, such as nitrous oxide and carbon monoxide, can interfere with the reading.

◆ Presence of nitrogen and nitrous oxide in the gas mixture can result in a collision broadening effect which increases the absorption of infrared light.

◆ A change in atmospheric pressure can affect the reading.

◆ Water moisture can affect the reading.

Total:	/20

Measurement of CO_2 tension

In 1954, Richard Stow described a CO_2 electrode using a rubber membrane permeable to CO_2 to separate a wet pH and reference electrode from a blood sample. Severinghaus modified this electrode stabilising it with a bicarbonate salt solution and a nylon mesh spacer.

The Severinghaus CO_2 electrode consists of two electrodes: a measuring electrode and a reference electrode. The measuring electrode consists of pH (H^+) sensitive glass in contact with a nylon mesh containing a bicarbonate buffer. A thin Teflon or silicone membrane permeable to CO_2 separates the blood sample from the electrode. CO_2 diffuses from the blood into the buffer and changes the pH. The quantity of hydrogen ion generated and the fall in pH is proportional to the partial pressure of CO_2.

The CO_2 electrode is calibrated by equilibrating the buffer with solutions of two known CO_2 concentrations.

For measurement of CO_2 from a gas mixture, refer to OSCE set 1, station 1.14.

Key points

- The CO_2 tension in a blood sample is measured using the Severinghaus electrode.
- The Severinghaus electrode is maintained at a temperature of 37°C.
- The accuracy depends on the integrity of the semi-permeable membrane.

Station 5.10 Resuscitation: pulseless electrical activity

Information for the candidate

You are on call and have been asked to attend urgently to a surgical ward. A 36-year-old female patient who underwent laparoscopic cholecystectomy an hour ago has collapsed.

Examiner's mark sheet

marks

Ensures safety of patient and self (safe to approach). 1 ☐

Confirms that the patient is unresponsive to verbal command by gently shaking the shoulders. 2 ☐

Correctly assesses airway and breathing, and confirms that the patient is not breathing, assessing the carotid pulse at the same time. 2 ☐

Calls for help (specifies a surgeon in addition to the crash team). 1 ☐

The crash trolley defibrillator has arrived. What would you do next?   2 □

Apply pads and assess rhythm.

The ECG monitor shows a heart rate of 65 per minute, sinus rhythm and no carotid pulse. What is this termed? What would you do next?   4 □

This patient has pulseless electrical activity (PEA); it is a non-shockable rhythm. Continue CPR in 2-minute cycles, secure an IV access, perform tracheal intubation, ventilate with 100% oxygen and give adrenaline 1mg every 3-5 minutes.

Now the blood pressure is 70 mm Hg systolic, the patient is breathing spontaneously

What are the reversible causes for pulseless electrical activity?   4 □

◆ Hypoxia, Hypovolaemia, Hyper and hypokalaemia and Hypothermia (4 Hs).
◆ Tension pneumothorax, cardiac Tamponade, Toxic (drug overdose) and Thrombus/pulmonary embolism (4Ts).

What is the most likely cause in this patient?   2 □

Severe hypovolaemia due to intra-abdominal bleeding.

During resuscitation this patient had 2L of warm Hartmann's solution. She appears very pale and her blood pressure is still low. What would be the next management?   2 □

Blood transfusion, surgical assessment and possible exploratory laparotomy.

Total: /20

Pulseless electrical activity

The presence of cardiac electrical activity (normal ECG complexes on the monitor) with the absence of palpable pulses is known as pulseless electrical activity (PEA). These patients have myocardial contractions, but not sufficient enough to produce cardiac output and a pulse.

PEA is often due to reversible causes (4Hs and 4Ts) and can be treated. The most common causes of cardiac arrest with PEA during the early postoperative period are haemorrhage and pulmonary embolism. However, other causes should be kept in mind.

After confirming the rhythm as PEA, CPR should be started at a 30:2 ratio (30 compressions: 2 breaths). If the rate is less than 60/minute, atropine 3mg should be given. If signs of life return during CPR, the rhythm and pulse should be checked. If the pulse is present post-resuscitation care should be provided. This includes immediate resuscitation with intravenous fluids, followed by blood transfusion if required.

If the rhythm changes to VF, it should be treated with defibrillation. If the rhythm persists to PEA, CPR should be continued and adrenaline 1mg should be given every 3-5 minutes.

In the event of a massive haemorrhage, the management strategies should include:

- Maintenance of circulation with resuscitation fluids.
- Improving oxygen-carrying capacity with blood transfusion.
- Surgical control of bleeding.

Key points

- PEA is often caused by reversible conditions and can be treated.
- Survival is unlikely unless the reversible cause is found and treated.
- If massive haemorrhage is suspected, obtaining surgical control of bleeding is essential.

Station 5.11 Anatomy: arterial system of the hand

Information for the candidate

In this station you will be asked questions on applied anatomy of the hand.

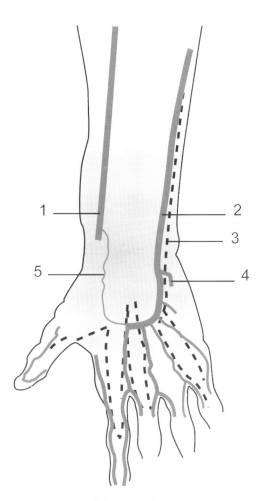

Figure 5.11 Arterial system of the hand.

Examiner's mark sheet

marks

Name the parts labelled 1-5 in Figure 5.11   5 ☐

1. Radial artery.
2. Ulnar artery.
3. Ulnar nerve.
4. Deep palmar branch of the ulnar artery.
5. Superficial palmar branch of the radial artery.

Which arteries can you cannulate in the forearm?   1 ☐

Radial, ulnar and brachial.

What precaution would you take before cannulating the radial artery?   1 ☐

Ensure that there is adequate ulnar collateral circulation in the hand.

What test would you do?   1 ☐

Allen's test.

What are the relations of the radial artery at the wrist?   2 ☐

It lies lateral to flexor carpi radialis and anterior to the pronator quadratus muscle and radius.

Describe the collateral circulation in the hand   3 ☐

The superficial and deep palmar arches provide collateral circulation in the hand. The ulnar artery continues as the superficial palmar arch and anastomoses with the superficial branch of the radial artery. The deep palmar arch of the radial artery anastomoses with a smaller deep branch of the ulnar artery.

How would you perform Allen's test? (Demonstrate on the actor)   4 ☐

- ◆ Elevate the hand and make a fist for 20 seconds.
- ◆ Then occlude both the ulnar and radial arteries.
- ◆ Open the fist and note that the hand is blanched white.
- ◆ Release the ulnar compression and note the flushing occurring within 5-10 seconds.

What are the complications of radial artery cannulation?   2 ☐

Infection, haematoma, thrombosis, distal ischaemia, embolisation, neurologic injury and pseudo-aneurysm.

Which nerve is more likely to be damaged?   1 ☐

The median nerve in the carpal tunnel is most likely to be compressed by a haematoma.

Total: /20

Arterial system of the hand

The ulnar artery enters the palm along the medial side of the wrist. It continues as the superficial palmar arch. The superficial palmar arch anastomoses with the superficial branch of the radial artery. The superficial palmar arch is covered by skin, the palmaris brevis muscle and the palmar aponeurosis.

The radial artery enters the hand along the lateral side of the wrist after crossing the anatomical snuffbox. It anastomoses with the deep branch of the ulnar artery to form the deep palmar arch.

Key points

◆ The radial artery is most commonly used for arterial cannulation. It is easily accessible and has a good collateral blood flow through the superficial palmar branch of the ulnar artery.

◆ Prior to cannulation the adequacy of the collateral circulation should be assessed using Allen's test (although the reliability of the test is questioned).

◆ The brachial artery is easily palpated medial to the biceps tendon. As it is the sole source of blood flow to the lower part of the forearm, thrombosis of the brachial artery can be catastrophic.

◆ Dorsalis pedis, posterior tibial and femoral arteries in the lower limb can be used for arterial cannulation.

Station 5.12 History taking: septoplasty

Information for the candidate

A 54-year-old male patient is scheduled to have a septoplasty. You will be asked to take a relevant history from the patient.

Examiner's mark sheet

marks

Introduces him/herself and confirms the nature of the proposed surgery.	2 ☐
Reason for proposed surgery (nasal obstruction).	1 ☐
Enquires as to whether the patient has been investigated for sleep apnoea.	2 ☐
Elicits symptoms related to obstructive sleep apnoea.	2 ☐

Station 5.13 Simulation: bronchospasm

Information for the candidate

A 30-year-old female patient who is a known asthmatic is on the operating table for an emergency appendicectomy. General anaesthesia was induced using a rapid sequence induction technique with thiopentone 250mg and suxamethonium 75mg. The laryngoscopic view was grade 1 and the trachea was easily intubated. Subsequently, atracurium 40mg and morphine 5mg were administered and the surgery has just begun.

On entering the station:

* Parameters on the monitor: SaO_2: 90%, HR: 78 per minute, BP: 130/80 mmHg.

* Airway pressure is high, end-tidal isoflurane: 0.9 in 40% oxygen and nitrous oxide.

Examiner's mark sheet

	marks	
Recognises increased airway pressure.	1	☐
Checks saturation, heart rate and blood pressure.	2	☐
Increases oxygen concentration.	2	☐
Hand ventilates and confirms the reduced compliance of the bag.	2	☐
Auscultates chest and identifies wheezing.	2	☐
Checks the endotracheal tube position/suctions the endotracheal tube.	2	☐
Increases the depth of anaesthesia.	1	☐

Administers a bronchodilator (nebulised salbutamol through a   2 ☐
catheter mount).

Asks for IV salbutamol or IV aminophylline.   2 ☐

Informs the surgeon and asks for help.   2 ☐

What is the dose of aminophylline?   1 ☐

5mg/Kg and maintenance is 0.5-0.9mg/Kg/hr.

What would you do if despite all the above measures   1 ☐
the patient is still wheezy and the saturation is 92%?

Administer adrenaline (epinephrine) 10µg IV bolus, increasing
up to 100µg in total.

Total:	/20

Information for the examiner

- Run the brochospasm scenario on the SimMan as the bell rings.
- Parameters on the monitor: SaO_2: 90%, HR: 78 per minute, BP: 130/80 mmHg.
- Airway pressure high, end-tidal isoflurane: 0.9 in 40% oxygen and nitrous oxide.
- Chest: bilateral wheezes and reduced compliance.

Intra-operative bronchospasm

This patient is a known asthmatic who has an increased risk of bronchospasm during the peri-operative period. As a result of bronchospasm, increased airway pressure is noted on the monitor (high pressure alarm on the ventilator is activated). You should immediately check the other vital parameters of the patient and then systematically investigate the cause of high airway pressure. Switching the ventilation to manual mode and hand ventilation helps to confirm the reduced compliance and rules out ventilator malfunction as a cause of high airway pressure. Visual inspection of the breathing system, including the breathing filter and catheter mount, should be carried out to exclude kinking and obstruction. Inspection and auscultation of the chest will aid you in diagnosing an intrathoracic cause of high airway pressure.

In severe bronchospasm, reduced air entry may lead to difficulty in differentiating from a tension pneumothorax. Tracheal deviation and a resonant note on percussion should aid in the diagnosis of a tension pneumothorax.

Management of bronchospasm

◆ Administer 100% oxygen.
◆ Stop respiratory irritant agents (e.g. desflurane) and increase the depth of anaesthesia using isoflurane or sevoflurane while maintaining haemodynamic stability.
◆ Exclude a breathing system or airway obstruction.
◆ Bronchodilators: a salbutamol inhaler, if immediately available, can be used in one of the following ways:
  ◦ disconnect the breathing system at the endotracheal end and discharge 2-4 puffs of salbutamol directly into the endotracheal tube, reconnect the system and ventilate. Most of the drug is likely to be deposited in the tracheal tube and can be inefficient;
  ◦ place the inhaler canister into the barrel of a 50ml leur lock syringe and replace the plunger. Attach the syringe to manometer tubing (infusion tubing) which is placed down the endotracheal tube and discharge 2-4 puffs by pressing the syringe plunger;
  ◦ using an appropriate T-piece adapter and external source of oxygen, 5mg of salbutamol can be nebulised into the breathing system between the breathing filter and endotracheal tube;
  ◦ intravenous salbutamol 250μg slow bolus followed by 5-10μg /minute infusion.
◆ Intravenous hydrocortisone 100mg.
◆ In extreme cases where there is no response to all the above measures, intravenous adrenaline may be used.

Key points

◆ Recognise the changes in vital parameters.
◆ Administer 100% oxygen.
◆ Increase the depth of anaesthesia if permitted by cardiovascular parameters.
◆ Administer inhaled (nebulised) or intravenous bronchodilators.

Station 5.14 Monitoring equipment: invasive blood pressure monitoring

Information for the candidate

In this station you will be expected to demonstrate your skills of setting up an invasive arterial blood pressure monitoring system.

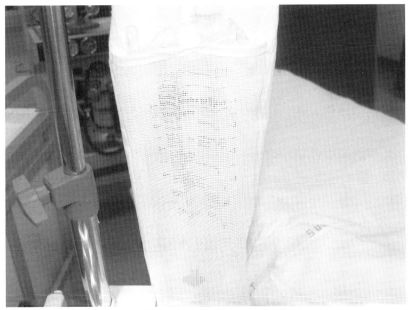

Figure 5.14a Intra-arterial blood pressure monitoring.

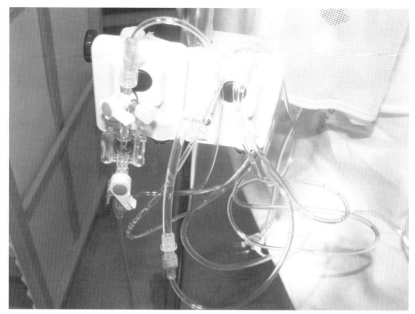

Figure 5.14b Intra-arterial blood pressure monitoring.

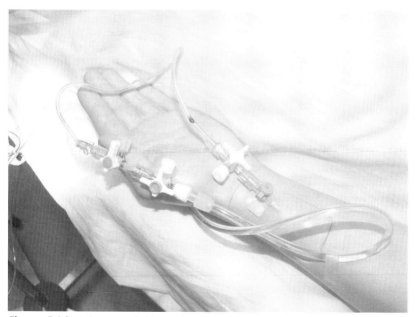

Figure 5.14c Intra-arterial blood pressure monitoring.

Examiner's mark sheet

marks

Check this arterial pressure monitoring system (in Figures 5.11a, 5.11b and 5.11c) and outline any faults

Infusion bag is not pressurised.   1 ☐

Transducer system is loosely attached.   1 ☐

Wrong catheter tubing (catheter tubing is not stiff).   1 ☐

Number of three-way stopcocks is more than required.   1 ☐

Arterial cannula (22G IV cannula) is too narrow for an adult patient.   1 ☐

What information can be obtained from an arterial waveform?
5 ☐

Heart rate, systolic and diastolic pressure, myocardial contractility, systemic vascular resistance and volume status (preload).

Describe how you would perform zero calibration of the transducer
2 ☐

The transducer is opened to the atmosphere by opening the three-way stopcock between the patient and transducer, and then selecting zero on the monitor.

How would you calibrate for a higher pressure?
2 ☐

The transducer is connected to an aneroid manometer using sterile tubing and the manometer pressure is raised to 100 and 200 mmHg. The monitor display should read the same pressure as the transducer.

Which of these is a normal arterial waveform? What is the problem with the other two? 3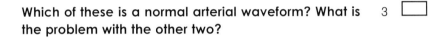

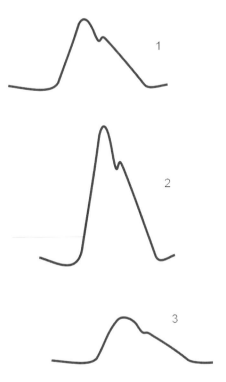

Figure 5.14d Arterial pressure waveforms.

(1) is normal, (2) is underdamped and (3) is an overdamped trace.

What will happen to the reading in a trace which is overdamped? 3

An overdamped trace under-reads systolic BP and over-reads diastolic BP; however, the mean blood pressure reading is not affected.

| Total: | /20 |

Invasive blood pressure monitoring

The arterial pressure monitoring system includes an arterial cannula, catheter tubing connecting the cannula to the transducer, a transducer, a pressurised flush system, a monitor to display the reading and waveform, and a cable connecting the transducer to the monitor. The purpose of the fluid-filled tubing system is to provide a means of transmitting the pressure generated in the artery to the transducer. Normal saline is used as the flushing fluid. The viscosity of the fluid used influences the natural frequency of the measurement system. Fluids with a viscosity higher than normal saline lead to overdamping. The flushing system is pressurised to 300 mmHg and provides a continuous slow flow of fluid (3-4ml/hr), preferably heparinised, to minimise the risk of clot formation in the catheter.

In order for the blood pressure waveform to be an accurate representation of the pressure within the artery, the column of fluid must convey the correct information to the strain gauge diaphragm. The arterial cannula should be wide and stiff. Increased compliance tends to reduce the natural frequency. The number of three-way taps should be kept to a minimum. Usually, one three-way stopcock is inserted between the arterial cannula and catheter tubing and another between the catheter tubing and transducer. Stopcocks have a narrower lumen than the catheter, therefore, they can reduce the natural frequency. The tubing system connecting the catheter to the transducer should be as short and as stiff-walled as possible, and free from bubbles and stopcocks.

An up-slope of the arterial waveform indicates myocardial contractility and a down-slope of the arterial waveform indicates systemic vascular resistance. Increased swing of the waveform during the respiratory cycle indicates a reduced preload.

Zero calibration eliminates the effect of atmospheric pressure on the measured pressure. To eliminate the gradient drift, calibration at a higher pressure is necessary. For accuracy, the transducer system must be 'zeroed' to a reference point, usually the level of the left ventricle, taken to be the mid-axillary line on the left side. Overdamping is usually produced by air bubbles, clots, catheter kinking, stopcocks, and narrow, compliant long tubing.

Key points

◆ For accurate measurement of arterial blood pressure, a measurement system with optimal damping is essential.
◆ A wide, short cannula with stiff tubing reduces the effect on damping.
◆ The number of stopcocks should be kept to a minimum as possible.
◆ Zero calibration eliminates the effect of atmospheric pressure on the measured pressure.
◆ An underdamped trace over-reads the systolic blood pressure and under-reads the diastolic blood pressure.

Station 5.15 Clinical safety: patient positioning

Information for the candidate

In this station your knowledge on the importance of positioning under anaesthesia and injuries pertaining to an improper position will be assessed.

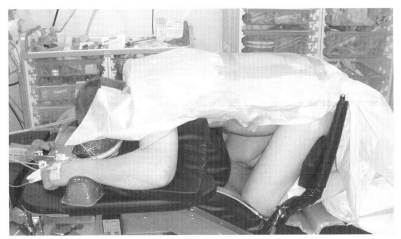

Figure 5.15a.

Examiner's mark sheet

marks

What is the position shown in Figure 5.15a?

1 ☐

Knee elbow position.

For what surgical procedures is this position used?

2 ☐

This position is used for posterior spinal decompression and laminectomy.

What are the problems associated with this position?

1 x 7 ☐
= 7

◆ Airway: endotracheal tube dislodgement, disconnection and kinking.
◆ Anatomical: nerve injury.
◆ Pressure effect on eyes and corneal abrasion.
◆ Soft tissue injury of the face (abrasion of nose, lips and cheeks).
◆ Skin ischaemia and subsequent ulcers over pressure points and bony prominences.
◆ Physiological: compression of femoral vessels resulting in an impaired venous return.
◆ Poor circulation and venous stasis in the lower limbs predisposing to deep vein thrombosis (DVT).

Which nerves can be injured and what is the mechanism?

2 x 5

=10

Table 5.15a Nerve injury.

Nerve involved	Mechanism of injury
Brachial plexus	Stretch due to excessive neck extension or shoulder rotation
Ulnar nerve	Direct pressure on the nerve
Peroneal nerve	Pressure over the head of the fibula
Lateral cutaneous nerve of the thigh	Pressure over the iliac crest by supporting poles
Supra-orbital nerve	Pressure from the head rest

Total: /20

Problems associated with patient positioning

Prone position

The prone position is used for surgery on the spine and spinal cord at the lumbar and thoracic regions. The trachea should be intubated with an armoured tracheal tube and should be firmly secured. The abdomen should be free to move so that ventilation is not impaired during the prone position. Care should be taken to prevent neurovascular injury. The neck and cervical spine should be kept in a neutral position during prone positioning. Excessive extension or flexion should be avoided. The forehead and face is supported using a soft jelly pad ring to minimise pressure effects.

In the simple prone position, the chest and pelvis should be supported with rolls or a Montreal mattress and care should be taken to allow enough room for diaphragmatic excursion and to prevent an increase in intra-abdominal pressure. Oedema of peri-orbital tissues is occasionally seen following the prone position.

Lateral position

The lateral position is used for total hip replacement and thoracotomy. The ulnar nerve, brachial plexus and the common peroneal nerve on the dependent side are vulnerable to injury.

Lithotomy position

The lithotomy position is used for urological and gynaecological procedures. Extreme flexion of the hips can compress the femoral nerve and vessels, and can stretch the sciatic nerve. The common peroneal nerve can be trapped between the head of the fibula and supporting stirrups. Pressure over the medial epicondyle of the tibia can result in saphenous nerve injury.

Lower limb compartment syndrome is a recognised complication of the lithotomy position, which results from a reduced perfusion of the lower limbs due to a prolonged lithotomy position.

Sitting position

The sitting position is used for posterior fossa surgery and shoulder surgery. The specific problems of this position include venous air embolism and postural hypotension. Excessive flexion of the neck can cause obstruction of carotid and vertebral arteries, leading to spinal cord ischaemia and stroke. Excessive extension or rotation of the neck and downward pull on the arms can result in brachial plexus injury. Knees should be flexed to avoid stretching of the sciatic nerve. Reduced venous return from the lower limbs can predispose to DVT.

Sensory deficit resulting from peripheral nerve injury (Figures 5.15b and 5.15c)

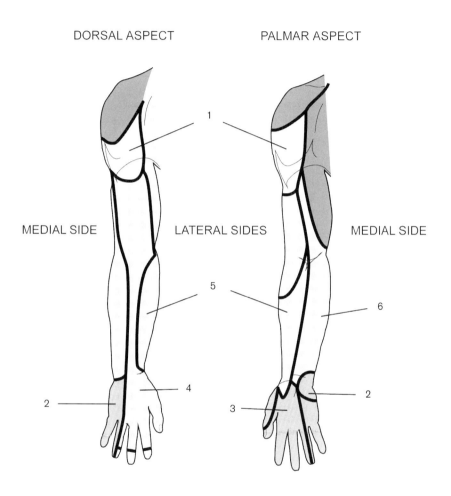

DORSAL ASPECT   PALMAR ASPECT

MEDIAL SIDE   LATERAL SIDES   MEDIAL SIDE

Figure 5.15b.

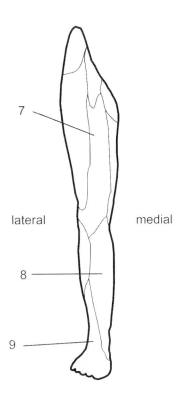

lateral   medial

Figure 5.15c.

Table 5.15b Nerve injury (numbers correspond to Figures 5.15b and c).

Nerve	Anatomical area of sensory deficit
1. Axillary	Over the lateral aspect of the shoulder
2. Ulnar	Little finger, medial half of the ring finger and medial third of the hand
3. Median	Palmar surface of the hand, lateral part of the ring finger, middle and index finger and thumb
4. Radial	Lateral aspect of the dorsum of the forearm and hand, thumb, index and middle fingers and lateral half of the ring finger on the dorsal aspect
5. Musculocutaneous	Radial aspect of the forearm
6. Medial cutaneous nerve of the forearm	Medial aspect of the forearm
7. Femoral	Anterior surface of the thigh up to the knee
8. Saphenous	Medial aspect of the knee, leg and foot
9. Common peroneal	Lateral aspect of the leg and dorsal surface of the foot

Peripheral nerve injuries of lower limb

(For peripheral nerve injuries of the upper limb, refer to OSCE set 4, station 4.15).

The sciatic nerve can be damaged by pressure against the hard surface of a table in a lateral position, a pneumatic tourniquet around the thigh with a pressure of more than 350 mm Hg and stretching of the nerve in a lithotomy position. Damage to the sciatic nerve at the level of the thigh will result in an inability to flex the knee joint. At the level of the knee joint, the sciatic nerve divides into two main terminal branches: the tibial nerve and common peroneal nerve. The common peroneal nerve is more vulnerable to damage as it passes around the head of the fibula. Damage results in foot drop and a loss of sensation over the lateral aspect of the leg and dorsum of the foot.

The femoral nerve is subject to damage at the level of the inguinal ligament and may be kinked in extreme flexion of the hip during a lithotomy position. Damage to the nerve at this level results in sensory loss over the anterior aspect of the thigh and an inability to extend the knee joint due to paralysis of the hamstring muscles.

The lateral cutaneous nerve of the thigh provides sensory supply over the lateral part of the lower gluteal region and anterolateral aspect of the thigh. Supporting frames used while the patient is in the prone position may damage the nerves. The saphenous nerve may be compressed against the medial tibial condyle if the legs are placed in a vertical stirrup support.

Key points

- A prone position is used for spinal decompression and for posterior cranial fossa surgery.
- Compression of the femoral vessels in a prone position may result in reduced venous return.
- Soft tissue injury of the face and pressure on the eyes should be avoided.

Station 5.16 Radiology: cervical spine X-ray

Information for the candidate

This is a cervical spine X-ray of a 69-year-old male patient who is scheduled for an emergency laparotomy. Two years ago he had fallen down from a ladder and sustained a neck injury. Six months ago he underwent an operative procedure on the cervical spine. A cervical spine X-ray, which was taken during pre-operative assessment, is presented. Inspect the cervical spine X-ray and answer the questions.

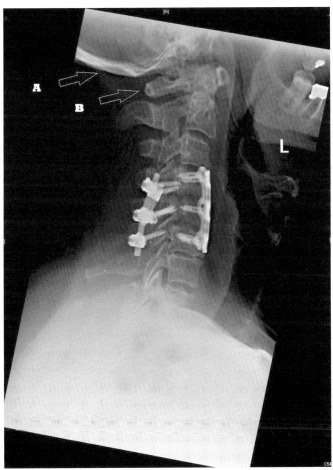

Figure 5.16 Cervical spine X-ray.

Examiner's mark sheet

Please tick the correct answer - true or false.   **marks**

1. There is malalignment of the vertebral bodies.   True   False   2 ☐
2. There is calcification of the anterior vertebral   True   False   2 ☐
   ligament.
3. All 7 cervical vertebrae are visualised in this X-ray. True   False   2 ☐
4. The space between the anterior arch of the atlas   True   False   2 ☐
   and odontoid process is increased.
5. The 3rd, 4th and 5th cervical vertebrae are fused   True   False   2 ☐
   using a plate and screws.
6. Rapid sequence intravenous induction can be   True   False   2 ☐
   performed safely.
7. Awake tracheal intubation is indicated in this   True   False   2 ☐
   patient.
8. The space between the anterior arch of the atlas   True   False   2 ☐
   and odontoid process of less than 3mm suggests
   atlanto-axial subluxation.
9. The gap between A and B is known as the atlanto-   True   False   2 ☐
   occipital gap.
10. An increased atlanto-occipital gap suggests a   True   False   2 ☐
    difficult intubation.

Total:	/20

Answers

1. True. There is malalignment at the level of the 2nd and 3rd vertebrae, as indicated by the line passing through the anterior vertebral bodies.

2. False.

3. False. The first three cervical vertebrae are clearly visible; the 4th, 5th and 6th vertebrae are fused using a plate and screws.

4. False. The space between the anterior arch of the atlas and the odontoid process is less than 3mm.

5. False. It is the 4th, 5th and 6th vertebrae which are fixed with a plate and screws.

6. False. This patient has a potentially difficult intubation.

7. True. This would be the safest plan for tracheal intubation in this patient.

8. False. A space between the anterior arch of the atlas and the odontoid process of more than 3mm suggests atlanto-axial subluxation, which may result in backward displacement of the odontoid process and compression of the spinal cord.

9. True. A is the occiput and B is the posterior process of the atlas. A reduced atlanto-occipital gap limits the extension of the head and results in a poor laryngoscopic view.

10. False.

Interpretation of the cervical spine X-ray

As with the chest X-ray, a systematic approach is used for reading the cervical spine X-ray. In a patient with a suspected cervical spine injury three views are necessary to exclude cervical spine injury:

*   Lateral view.
*   Anteroposterior view.
*   Open mouth odontoid view.

A lateral cervical spine X-ray should include all 7 vertebrae and the upper half of the first thoracic vertebra. An open mouth odontoid view involving the odontoid process and lateral mass of the atlas (C1) is useful in diagnosing fracture or lateral displacement of the odontoid process.

A systematic approach includes the following:

A: Alignment of the cervical spine is assessed using 4 lordotic curves:

- A line passing through the anterior vertebral bodies.
- A line passing through the anterior aspect of the spinal canal.
- A line passing through the posterior aspect of the spinal canal.
- A line passing through the tips of the spinous processes.

B: Bony components of the cervical spine are assessed by observing the contour, height of the vertebral body, pedicle, laminae, and the transverse and spinous processes.

C: The cartilaginous area includes the intervertebral discs and the posterolateral facet joints. Vertebral malalignment of more than 3mm suggests vertebral dislocation. A reduction in anterior height of the vertebral body of more than 3mm suggests a compression fracture.

Soft tissue contour: in suspected cases of cervical spine injury prominence of the pre-vertebral soft tissue shadow in front of the line passing through the anterior vertebral bodies indicates haemorrhage. Soft tissue thickness anterior to C2 should be less than 6mm and anterior to C4-C7 should be less than 20-22mm.

Key points

- A lateral cervical spine X-ray should include all 7 vertebrae and the upper half of the first thoracic vertebra.
- Lucency through the tip of the odontoid process suggests fracture.
- A normal space between the anterior arch of the atlas and the odontoid process is less than 3mm.
- Vertebral malalignment of more than 3mm suggests vertebral dislocation.

Station 5.17 History taking: abdominal hysterectomy

Information for the candidate

In this station you will be asked to take a history from a 48-year-old female patient scheduled to have an abdominal hysterectomy

Examiner's mark sheet

marks

Introduces him/herself to the patient, confirming that he/she is talking to the right person and explains his/her role.　2 ☐

H/O previous anaesthetic: PONV following dental extraction.　2 ☐

Current presentation: per-vaginal bleeding.　1 ☐

Palpitations and shortness of breath on climbing a flight of stairs.　2 ☐

H/O anaemia.　2 ☐

H/O migraine.　1 ☐

H/O DVT, pulmonary embolism 6 months ago.　2 ☐

Drug history: warfarin.　1 ☐

Specifically asks for dose and logbook (yellow) for INR.　2 ☐

Other regular drugs

Ibuprofen for migraine.　1 ☐
Iron tablets for anaemia.　1 ☐

H/O allergy: none known.　1 ☐

H/O smoking: 20 cigarettes a day.　1 ☐

H/O alcohol intake: none.   1 ☐

Total: /20

Information for the actor

You are a 48-year-old female scheduled to have a hysterectomy (removal of the womb). You have suffered from vaginal bleeding for the past year secondary to some new growths (fibroids) in the uterus. Consequent to the blood loss, you are quite anaemic (reduced red cells in blood). Nowadays, you get tired, have shortness of breath and palpitations even after climbing up a flight of stairs. Your GP has started you on iron tablets.

Six months ago you developed severe pain and swelling in your left calf and subsequently suffered tightness of the chest. You were diagnosed with deep vein thrombosis (clot in the leg) and pulmonary embolism (clot in the lung). Since then you were started on a medicine, warfarin, which prevents clot formation, but can cause bleeding. You have a little yellow book to follow-up with your doctor in which the details of the medicine dosage and clotting are entered on a regular basis.

Some years ago you underwent teeth extraction under general anaesthesia and were admitted to hospital after the procedure for severe nausea and vomiting. You suffer from migraine for which you take ibuprofen. You have no known allergies to medicine or food. You smoke about 20 cigarettes a day, but do not consume alcoholic beverages.

Anticoagulation with warfarin

Patients can be given warfarin either for venous or for arterial thrombo-embolic diseases. Venous thrombo-embolism conditions include deep vein thrombosis (DVT), pulmonary embolism (PE), and deficiencies of antithrombin III, protein C and protein S. Arterial thrombo-embolism conditions include atrial fibrillation, acute myocardial infarction, mural cardiac thrombus, and problems associated with prosthetic heart valves.

The effect of warfarin is monitored by measuring the INR. In treatment of DVT, PE, atrial fibrillation, patients with tissue heart valves, and valvular heart disease, a therapeutic range of INR of 2.0-3.0 is recommended. In the presence of mechanical prosthetic valves or recurrent systemic emboli, the recommended range is 2.5-3.5.

In the peri-operative period, the decision to continue or withhold warfarin is determined by balancing the risks of recurring thrombo-embolism and surgical bleeding. In general, warfarin is stopped 3-5 days prior to surgery. If the risk of thrombo-embolism is high, in the absence of a warfarin effect, patients should receive 'heparin bridging' with unfractionated or low-molecular-weight heparin until warfarinisation is re-established. Seeking a haematologist's advice will be valuable.

Key points

- ◆ Use a structured approach.
- ◆ Explore the reason for the proposed surgery.
- ◆ If patients volunteer a history of conditions, such as anaemia, explore more about its systemic effects.
- ◆ Do not forget to elicit a history of exercise tolerance.
- ◆ Ask details about the drugs and the reason for taking the drugs.

(For more information please refer to OSCE set 1, station 1.12).

Station 5.18 Communication: abdominal aortic aneurysm repair

Information for the candidate

A 70-year-old man underwent emergency repair of a ruptured abdominal aortic aneurysm. Intra-operative blood loss was 3.5L; 8 units of blood were transfused during the surgery. An arterial blood gas shows severe metabolic acidosis. He is ventilated in the intensive care unit. He requires an adrenaline infusion at a rate of 0.4mg per hour.

In this station you will meet the patient's son.

Examiner's mark sheet

marks

Introduces him/herself to the patient's relative.   1   ☐

Ensures that the relative is able to understand the role of the abdominal aorta (as a major blood vessel) and the consequences of a leaking or ruptured aneurysm.   1   ☐

Elicits relative's understanding and details already known to the relative.   2   ☐

Explains the nature of the surgery and the reason for doing the surgery.   2   ☐

Explains the nature and seriousness of the problem in simple terms.   1   ☐

Explains about intra-operative blood loss and blood transfusion.   2   ☐

Explains the reason for ventilating.   2   ☐

Reassures that he is sedated and pain is controlled.   2   ☐

Gives details about the current general condition.   2   ☐

Gives details on possible complications that can be anticipated in the next 24-48 hours.   2   ☐

Ensures that the relative understands the seriousness of the problem and associated mortality.   2   ☐

Gives an opportunity for further questions and clarification.   1   ☐

Total: /20

Information for the actor

Your father (70 years old) is admitted to the hospital and you have been told that he is seriously ill. You visited him a week ago and he seemed fine. You know that he has mild diabetes and high blood pressure. He has neither been admitted to hospital in the past, nor had any operations. You have no idea what this emergency operation was for.

Your concerns are: How is he? Can you see him? When will he be able to go home? Did he receive the right treatment? Can you speak to the senior surgeon who operated on him? The doctor may mention that he is on a breathing machine which will make you worried that his condition may be serious.

Communication skill: providing information to the patient's relative

Convey the facts to the relative who may not have any background knowledge about the patient's illness. The pathology and illness should be explained in simple language. Issues such as major surgery, pre-operative comorbidity, postoperative complications and mortality should be outlined to the relative or next of kin.

Have a list of simple layman words for complex medical terminology. An example for the abdominal aorta would be: a major blood pipe inside the tummy; for the ventilator: a breathing machine; and for the endotracheal tube: a breathing tube to the windpipe.

A ruptured aortic aneurysm has a high mortality rate (nearly 50%). Intra-operative blood loss, problems related to blood transfusion, hypotension, reduced organ perfusion, aortic cross-clamping - all contribute to increased peri-operative morbidity. The majority of patients require intra-operative inotropic support. Renal failure, myocardial infarction, continued bleeding and retroperitoneal bleeding, pulmonary embolism, and graft infection are the major complications during the postoperative period.

Key points

◆ Convey the facts sensitively.
◆ Establish the understanding and knowledge of the relative about the patient.
◆ A ruptured aortic aneurysm has a high mortality rate.

Station 5.19 Anatomy: spine and vertebrae

Information for the candidate

In this station you will be asked questions on anatomy and the technical skill required for performing epidural anaesthesia.

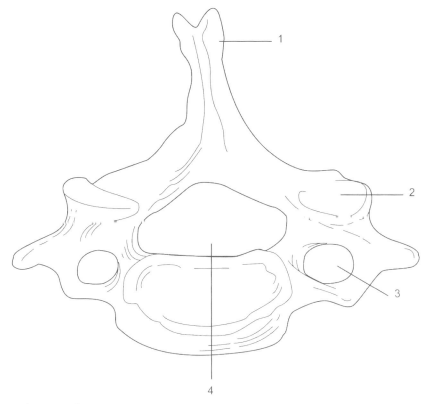

Figure 5.19a.

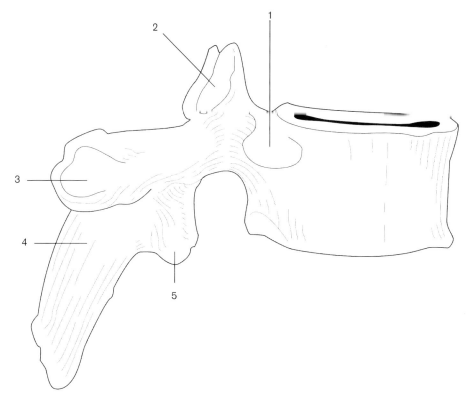

Figure 5.19b.

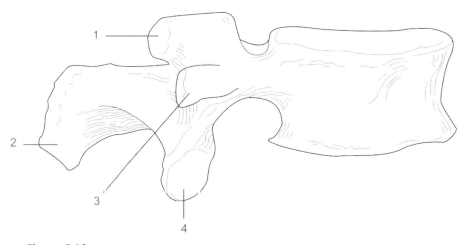

Figure 5.19c.

Examiner's mark sheet

marks

Name the vertebrae in Figures 5.19a, 5.19b and 5.19c   3 ☐

- ◆ Figure 5.19a: typical cervical vertebra.
- ◆ Figure 5.19b: typical thoracic vertebra.
- ◆ Figure 5.19c: typical lumbar vertebra.

Figure 5.19a

1. Spinous process.
2. Superior articular facet.
3. Foramen transversarium.
4. Vertebral foramen.

Figure 5.19b

1. Facet for rib attachment.
2. Superior articular facet.
3. Transverse process.
4. Spinous process.
5. Inferior articular process.

Figure 5.19c

1. Superior articular process.
2. Spinous process.
3. Transverse process.
4. Inferior articular process.

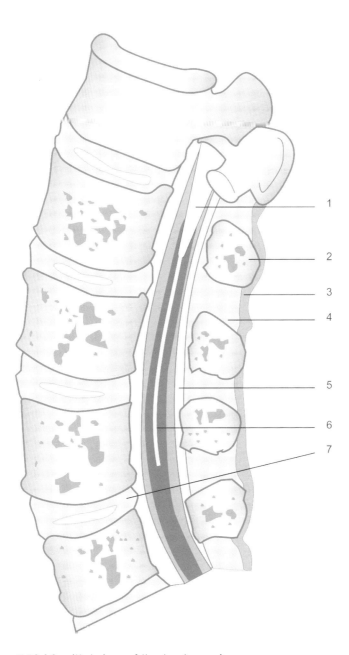

Figure 5.19d Sagittal view of the lumbar spine.

Name the structures labelled 1 to 6 in Figure 5.19d   6 ☐

1. Spinal cord.
2. Spinous process.
3. Supraspinous ligament.
4. Interspinous ligament.
5. Ligamentum flavum.
6. Filum terminale.
7. Intervertebral disc.

What are the differences between thoracic and lumbar vertebrae?   2 ☐

Thoracic vertebrae have the following features (refer to Figure 5.19b):

◆ Upper and lower hemi-facets (on the body) for the attachment of rib heads.
◆ The transverse processes are larger than lumbar vertebrae.
◆ The transverse process has a facet which articulates with the tubercle of the rib.
◆ Spinous processes are long and angulate downwards; lumbar spinous processes are horizontal and are perpendicular to the body of the vertebra.

You are asked to perform an epidural block at the L1-L2 interspace. Can you describe the procedure?   6 ☐

◆ Preparation: ensures that the patient has been consented and all drugs and equipment are available and checked.
◆ Mentions aseptic precautions.
◆ Selects appropriate position.
◆ Correctly locates L1-2 interspace (on an actor).
◆ Describes:
  • preparation of back with antiseptic solution;
  • local anaesthetic injection to skin and deeper tissues;
  • appropriate technique to identify the epidural space.

How much of the catheter would you insert into the space? 1 ☐

About 4-5cm of catheter should be left in the space.

Would you use a test dose? What is the purpose of a test dose? 2 ☐

A test dose of 10mg of bupivacaine is used to identify the subarachnoid placement of the catheter.

Total:	/20

Epidural anaesthesia

The epidural space is a potential space that lies between the dura and periosteum lining the inner aspect of the vertebral canal. On the posterior aspect the ligamentum flavum completes the boundary between the laminae. It extends from the foramen magnum to the sacral hiatus. It contains fat, areolar tissue and a vertebral venous plexus.

The line joining the top of the iliac crests usually corresponds to the level of the L4 vertebra. The space just above the line is usually the L3-L4 inter-space. The epidural space can be identified by either using a loss of resistance technique or negative pressure technique.

With the loss of resistance method, a syringe filled either with saline or air is used to locate the epidural space. The disadvantages of air include the potential for injection of air into the vascular space and subarachnoid space (pneumocephalus), and the greater incidence of the catheter puncturing the epidural veins. Saline tends to push the dura away from the needle tip as it enters the epidural space.

Negative pressure techniques, such as a visual indication of pressure change, sucking in of a hanging drop or sucking in of fluid from a drip attached to the epidural needle, have been used.

The use of a test dose is still a controversial practice. A test dose cannot reliably identify the intravascular placement of a catheter. But 10mg of bupivacaine injected into the subarachnoid space will produce some motor block.

Key points

♦ Epidural technique involves preparation of the patient (assessment, consent), preparation of theatre (trained assistant, drugs, equipment), preparation of the site (positioning, aseptic precautions) and then performance of the block.
♦ The intercristal line corresponds to the L4 vertebra.
♦ More than 5cm of the catheter in the epidural space can exit through the intervetebral foramen causing a unilateral block; less than 4cm poses a risk of accidental dislodgement. The optimal recommended length in the epidural space is 4-5cm.

Station 5.20 Technical skill: supraclavicular brachial plexus block

Information for the candidate

In this station you will be asked questions to assess your knowledge and skills related to supraclavicular brachial plexus block.

Examiner's mark sheet

marks

Describe the relations of the brachial plexus in the neck   4   ☐

The brachial plexus is formed by the union of the anterior primary rami of the lower 4 cervical nerves and the anterior primary rami of the first thoracic nerve (C5-T1). The roots emerge from the intervertebral foramina. The roots of the 5th and 6th cervical nerves unite to form the upper trunk. The root of the 7th cervical nerve continues as the middle trunk. The 8th cervical nerve and 1st thoracic nerve roots unite to form the lower trunk.

In the neck the roots and trunks lie in the posterior triangle, covered by skin, platysma and deep fascia. Superficially the plexus is crossed by the external jugular vein and the supraclavicular nerves. The trunks emerge from the space between the scalenus anterior and scalenus medius muscles. This space becomes wider in the anteroposterior plane as the muscles approach their insertion on the first rib. The plexus leaves the neck by crossing the clavicle near its midpoint.

What are the indications for supraclavicular brachial plexus block?   2 ☐

A supraclavicular brachial plexus block can be used as a sole anaesthetic technique or as a supplement to general anaesthesia for surgeries in the shoulder, arm and forearm.

Describe the technique of performing the supraclavicular block   2 ☐

- ◆ Preparation: ensure that the patient has been consented and that all drugs, equipment and monitors are available and checked; use aseptic precautions.
- ◆ Position: head slightly turned to the opposite side.

Indicate the landmarks and point of needle entry (on the actor)   4 ☐

The midpoint of the clavicle is located midway between the acromial end and sternal end of the clavicle. The point of needle entry is 1cm above the midclavicular point, lateral to the insertion of the clavicular head of sternocleidomastoid and lateral to the subclavian artery pulsation.

The skin is infiltrated with 1ml of 1% lidocaine. An insulated nerve stimulator needle is inserted perpendicular to the skin. Using a nerve stimulator, contractions of the forearm muscles can be observed. Once muscle contractions are elicited at a current of less than 0.5mA, 30-40ml of local anaesthetic can be injected following careful negative aspiration.

What part of the brachial plexus would you stimulate with this approach? 2 ☐

The trunk of the brachial plexus is stimulated at this level. The plexus is quite close at this region. A dense block is often possible in this approach.

What are the contra-indications for this block? 4 ☐

General contra-indications for the nerve block include patient refusal, allergy to local anaesthetics, bleeding disorders and infection at the site.

Specific relative contra-indications for supraclavicular block are a short, stiff neck, large goitre, previous radiotherapy to the neck, previous radical neck surgery and recurrent laryngeal nerve palsy, and a pneumothorax in the opposite side.

What movements are elicited when you stimulate i) the lateral cord and ii) the posterior cord? 2 ☐

- Stimulation of the lateral cord causes the contraction of biceps with elbow flexion (musculocutaneous nerve).
- Stimulation of the posterior cord causes contraction of triceps and elbow extension (radial nerve).

Total: /20

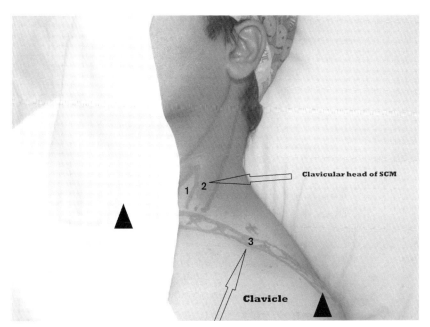

Figure 5.20 Landmarks for supraclavicular brachial plexus block.
1. Sternal head of sternocleidomastoid; 2. Clavicular head of sternocleidomastoid; 3. Midpoint of the clavicle.

Use of a nerve stimulator to locate the nerves

Use of the nerve stimulator increases the success of peripheral nerve blocks. It provides objective evidence that the needle tip is close to the nerve. Using a short square wave impulse of 0.1 msec duration, only the motor fibres can be stimulated without stimulating the C-fibres. Hence, it does not cause pain.

Insulating the needles except for the tip reduces dispersion of current; hence, insulated needles require less current. The cathode (negative electrode) causes depolarisation of the nerve, therefore requiring less current to stimulate the nerve. The anode causes an area of hyper-polarisation around the needle and requires a higher current to stimulate the nerve. A stimulating frequency of 2Hz is usually chosen. A high frequency causes painful muscle twitches. If the frequency of stimulation is too slow, the nerve may be impaled. If a muscle twitch is generated at very low current of less than 0.2mA, there is a possibility that the needle may penetrate the nerve.

Once the appropriate twitch is generated, maintaining the immobility of the needle, 1ml of local anaesthetic is injected. This causes mechanical displacement of the nerve away from the needle tip and results in the immediate disappearance of the twitches.

Key points

◆ Stimulation of the radial nerve (C7, C8) elicits extension of the elbow, wrist and finger.
◆ Stimulation of the ulnar nerve (C8, T1) elicits wrist flexion and medial deviation.
◆ Stimulation of the median nerve (C5-8) elicits wrist flexion, finger flexion and thumb opposition.